WEED INKED

DEDICATION

To the Wolf, the Gambler and the Dragon.
Because I said I would.

AKNOWLEDGMENTS

I stand on the shoulders of giants. So many have done the real work researching over the years and we are all grateful.

Dr. Latisha Bader not only contributed a key chapter but encourages me to keep growing and learning. She is a remarkable contributor to this discussion and a dear friend.

Issy Simpson approached me several years ago at an event for student athletes, she is a hell of a golfer and played for CU. For an exceptionally bright person and future world leader, Issy made a very questionable decision when we spoke and offered to help me in my work, poor girl. Issy did the research for this book and I didn't make it easy on her but she did it expertly. She made my work doable, this book would not exist without her. You will do great things Issy, thank you for all your amazing help.

Jamie Millin has what is arguably the worst job on earth, she has to get me where I'm supposed to be and poke and prod me into doing all of the things I overcommitted to doing. I would never finish anything, ever, like anything, were it not for Jamie's 24/7 support.

Charlie Bentz is my partner in several ventures and a consistent source of encouragement. Thank you for pushing me Charlie and for your notes on the early drafts.

Les Lefthand has allowed me to be a part of his community inside of The Crow Nation and has taught me much about spirituality and recovery. I just wish he could have done so in sweat lodges that were a bit less hot.

Dr. Kevin Sabet continues to be the nations, and really the worlds thought leader on this subject. I'm grateful for his help, encouragement and mostly his friendship.

Chris Carlough fights for sobriety and mental health like a soldier who burned the ships, he inspires me.

Tom Walker is always there for me, even when he really doesn't want to be.

Kris Washington has the eye for design that I never will and his understanding of this discussion makes that insight invaluable.

Steve Cort to most, Dad to a few of us. Thanks for all of your help on this project. I know how smart you are so you obviously learned your lesson on the first book but still offered to edit this one as well. Not only was your work extremely helpful, it was a lot of fun doing this with you.

Christy, the only other person on earth who understands: Fight for it, you will come out on top. Tomorrow is a new day you should begin it well and serenely.

The warriors who continue to fight the good fight, those who are not intimidated by loud voices trying to speak over their truth....

Sally Schindel, Laura Stack, Dawn Reinfeld, Aubree Adams, Luke Niforatos, Patrick Kennedy, Rhea Parsons, Karen Sylvester, Monte Stiles, SMART Colorado, SAM and The Foundation For Drug Policy Solutions, Dr. Roneet Lev, Dr. Libby Stout, Kim Porter, Jo McGuire, Dr. Ken Finn.

ABOUT THE AUTHOR

It occurs to me, as it should to you, that I self-published this book so I can spin any load of BS about myself that I want! Rest assured dear reader; I would never consider doing anything like that…

Ben received his first master's degree at age 13 and went on to achieve 4 more prior to getting his PhD at 19 followed by his MD at 21, much like Doogie Howser. Ben holds the current shot-put record for men over 45 weighing less than 250 lbs. Ben is a competitive F1 driver for both Mercedes and Ferrari, often racing for both in the same event.

In everyone else's reality; Ben barely made it out of high school and was almost of legal age to buy beer when he finally did. He sobered up early which allowed him to get that much coveted diploma.

He went on to 'pursue a career' in manual labor which was cut short due to injury forcing him to sit at a desk for his minimum wage. While Ben's current peers were getting degrees and advanced degrees Ben caught a lot of fish on his fly-rod and climbed a bunch of rock and ice. These activities led him to his real claim to fame, the breaking of 34 bones, not including fingers and toes of course. Keep his 11 diagnosed concussions in mind while reading, he really is trying, bless his heart.

He joined the field in 2007 when he was 11 years sober and now runs several companies, all related to behavioral health, that are successful only because he is good at hiring people who are much smarter than he is.

In addition to those companies Ben speaks live to about 20k people a year on this and similar subjects. He assists multiple collegiate athletic programs as well as professional athletic teams with crisis management and education for substance abuse and addiction. All these work activities keep getting in the way of his fishing but seeing the magic that is recovery and being able to help in some of life's most desperate moments makes that worth it.

He also gave a TEDx talk that got picked up by TED and featured as the talk of the week that a bunch of people watched. He thinks numbers of clicks and social media are silly.

His beat up old body tolerates fishing and some archery hunting but not much else when he isn't working. If one can read too much Ben probably does.

FORWARD

It is with great pleasure and enthusiasm that I introduce to you the captivating and thought-provoking book *Weed Inked*. *Weed, Inked* is a follow-up to Ben's first book, published in 2017 called *Weed, Inc.: The Truth About the Pot Lobby, THC, and the Commercial Marijuana Industry*. This book is updated with facts, figures, and brilliant illustrations.

In a world where cannabis use is becoming increasingly prevalent, it is essential to address the potential risks and negative consequences associated with its consumption. *Weed, Inked* provides such insight and information. Whether you are personally struggling with weed addiction, concerned about a loved one, or simply curious about the topic, this book will provide you with the insights, information, and guidance you need.

This volume does not pass judgment or criticize those who choose to use cannabis. Instead, it aims to provide a well-researched and informative resource and is a culmination of years of research, expert insights, and personal experiences, all aimed at shedding light on the physical, mental, and social impacts of cannabis use.

In the book, Ben stresses the need for using more accurate language (high potency THC vs CBD based medications) and dealing with the harms of this potent form of THC. He discusses the mental and physical health effects of high potency THC and the market forces behind them and how it boils down to another "addiction for profit" industry, like big tobacco industry. *Weed, Inked* is basically an indictment of the commercial cannabis industry.

Ben is my go-to guy for information on cannabis, CBD, and marijuana laws. He's also a consummate clinician, public speaker, educated administrator and a heck of a storyteller. This book reads like an expose and that's what it is. The information is up to date and Ben knows the topic inside and out. He has been on the forefront of this issue not as some anti-drug warrior, but rather as a concept translator who pushes common sense rather than reactive and shallow thinking.

Almost 40 years ago, I stopped using mood -altering drugs and entered a 12-step support group for, you guessed it, "weed" (which we called "grass" in those days). I was stoned every day for 12 years, and simply couldn't stay stopped till I truly sobered up in a mutual help group, specifically AA. It astounds me to realize that the potency now, compared to then is increased astronomically. For me, the drug led to dangerous activities, low motivation, downright sloth, weight gain, and dulled cognition. If I used the products described in this book, I fear I wouldn't be around to write this note.

Furthermore, as an addiction specialist for over 40 years, I've seen the trends described here – increased potency and increase in dire consequences, the most concerning being severe anxiety disorders and psychosis. Just recently a study in the International Journal of Drug Policy found an increased prevalence of violent behavior among males reporting daily cannabis use with and without cannabis use disorder (CUD) versus no cannabis use. Violence and psychosis related to cannabis use go hand in hand in my clinical experience.

Here are some sobering facts from a recent summary article by my colleague, Mark Gold, MD in Psychology Today which highlight the concerns raised in the book:

- Young adults and teens can develop an addiction to weed and become psychotic.

- Many people don't know that regular marijuana use may carry serious health risks, especially for the young.

- No medication is FDA-approved for treating cannabis use disorder.

- One cannabis-induced psychotic episode ups the risk of developing bipolar disorder or schizophrenia by 50%.

As of March 2024, 24 states have legalized recreational marijuana for individuals aged 21 years and older. As support for legalization increases, concerns remain that it will encourage marijuana use in young people. Youth marijuana use has been associated with adverse health outcomes and poorer academic performance.

The financial realities of the cannabis industry are staggering and eye-opening. Cannabis businesses earned $37 billion in 2023 and are projected to double by 2030. This, like the tobacco industry are the worst examples of corporate greed at the expense of the well-being of our children.

A few of the most cogent direct quotes from "Weed, Inked" include:

High potency "concentrates have no place in the human brain or body, none. There is ample proof that they are unsafe and there exists no evidence that they are in any way safe. Yet they have a huge place in the commercial market."

"For-profit sales lead to a focus on the frequent user, the frequent user builds tolerance, and tolerance demands stronger products; a market in which concentrates rule."

"By sanctioning another intoxicating and addictive substance, and worst of all by failing to regulate it, we see another unfortunate and dangerous demonstration of profit over people".

"If it can be introduced into the human body, someone is infusing it with THC and selling it, often with kids in mind. This is an issue for several reasons, the most obvious concerns how easy these products are to conceal and use in plain sight. Think of kids in school; few administrators are looking for the THC infused lollipops."

By this point, I found that my jaw had dropped, and I felt like I was descending a dark hole. The cannabis industry is a huge concern for all of us.

Some of the potential drawbacks of legalizing cannabis include:

- Health Risks: (impaired cognitive function, increased risk of addiction, respiratory problems, and mental health issues in vulnerable individuals).

- Increased Availability leading to higher levels of use, especially among young people, in view of perceived sense of safety of the drug.

- Road Safety: from the increased incidence of impaired driving.

- Regulatory Challenges: Developing effective regulations and enforcement mechanisms for the cannabis industry are complex and require a considerable investment of resources.

According to the CDC, 22% of Americans 12 years of age or older, or 19 million people, used cannabis in 2022, with highest usage among those 18-25 years old (38%). In 2022, 30.7% of twelfth graders reported using cannabis in the past year, and *6.3% used cannabis daily in the past 30 days.*

Cannabis use disorder (CUD) is also increasing; in 2022, 5.7 million people met diagnostic criteria for this disorder. The risk was highest (16.5%) among young adults ages 18-25. The core feature of the disorder is that users can't stop using even though cannabis causes adverse consequences. Some people with CUD smoke marijuana multiple times every day.

In a world where the acceptance and accessibility of cannabis are on the rise, *Weed, Inked* is a welcome vehicle for the reader to be able address the potential risks and consequences associated with its consumption in an informed manner.

-Mel Pohl, MD, DFASAM

CONTENTS

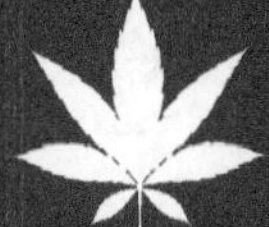

CHAPTER

01

TOLD YA SO

Why it might be a good idea to pay attention this time and what's coming next

When people find out, that you're writing a book, the first question is often the same; "What's the title?" I never know what to say because if this is anything like the last one the title will be three changes from the one I suggested because, I guess, publishers know best, or whatever. Thankfully the title I hoped for made it and led to the creation of the super cool cover you just turned. My wife and the editor pointed out that my skills in subtlety lack clarity, so a little explanation.

The last book was called Weed Inc, so this is totally witty, I just added two letters! The real idea is how we basically tattooed weed on the forearm of our country, and it was a bad tattoo, it's not going to age well, like the guys from the service fifty years ago whose ship name now looks like a black blob. We don't get tattoos of other drugs, except maybe booze and my friend 'Jailbird Joe,'a childhood friend who had 'THC' prison tattooed on his arm. Weed enjoys a place in the American mind that other drugs simply don't. What I hope to prove to the reader is why this was a mistake.

"When are you going to write another book?" they ask

My answer, "Never, the last one was way too much of a pain in my ass!"

That was, of course, until I started doing the math and seeing all of the dollar signs $$$$$$, If I were to add up all I made from WEED Inc vs the time it took to write I had to have made a solid $1/hr! Seriously, to you young idealists out there: don't become a writer, you will die hungry.

If it isn't for the money then why write another? The fame? Can't check that box either, I'm not into that nonsense. I really respect the singer Sia and how she rolls. She wears a mask or a wig that hides her face to maintain privacy. If I could do everything publicly that I do in one of my stylin COVID masks I would. More than anything I just want to hang out with my family, fish and do my work helping addicts find sobriety. I'm not into the spotlight.

A couple of years ago, after the first book, I gave a TEDx talk in Denver. TEDx isn't really a big deal, maybe a few thousand people saw it. But later the talk got picked up by the main TED stage and featured as their "talk of the day" for a while which has led to better than 4 million views, the majority of which I still believe are my mother showing everyone she meets. It was and is outside of my comfort zone to be that far out front.

If not for the notoriety, maybe I am writing because my art needs to breathe, I have to create? Nope, not that either. As you are already realizing, or know from the first book, I'm really not that good at this writing business. I write fun short stories that I share only with my wife, and sometimes kids, if they aren't too dark. I'm not a very good author.

My wife is a brilliant artist, a painter and poet, she creates beauty and loves those mediums, neither really speak to me. For me literature is humanities highest form of art. I am somewhat embarrassed to be introducing more mediocre literature into an overcrowded shelf.

So why another book? Simple, there are some things that you need to understand about weed and what's going on, and this is the most efficient way of getting the information out since I don't mess with social media. Things have changed since Weed Inc was published in 2017 and we need to understand more than we currently do as a society. We continue to have discussions about something that is not the thing being consumed. This reality is leading to some shortsighted lawmaking and much more pain then we need to deal with. We better understand what is actually happening as opposed to what the profiteers are telling us is taking place so we can find some balance. We need to understand the risks and rewards associated with cannabis, and all of its various forms and components which will allow us to make informed and insightful decisions, something I still have to hope that this crazy divided nation is capable of doing.

We are so damn polarized right now, and this issue is no exception. People tend to be all for or all opposed, and whenever we stand on dogma we are bound to miss some common sense. Or they are passive and avoid anything challenging by saying 'we should all just get along' and never engage in real conversation. PLEASE, try to consider the following pages without the filter you bring to this issue; cannabis is neither a panacea nor is it the devils lettuce. Those saying otherwise are selling something. I began the last book with a similar warning: If you are so entrenched in your belief system on this topic this book isn't for you. I do not have the skill or patience to reverse anyone's fundamental belief system, I hope to challenge some of what you might think or believe, but these words will fall on deaf ears if you are locked into your narrative of this complex subject. This is not a republican vs democrat issue, it is not a black and white up or down conversation. This is more complicated and deserves more thought than that.

With that in mind, let me say again that I have no issue with the casual adult consumer of cannabis and its derivatives. My hope is that those of you who choose to consume do so with knowledge and understanding and can realistically weigh the risks and rewards which will allow you to move forward responsibly. Again, don't drive high and don't let kids see you.

My beef is with the industry and the individuals of that industry making billions each year ($27 billion in 2022). They are recklessly selling products that promote addiction, damage minds and bodies, hurt communities, cost us money and they pretend that they are in it for the good of all.[1] These guys, and they are almost all guys, have somehow gotten a pass from the scrutiny that we apply to other industries. To question weed and the claims made by those selling it are off limits in many circles. I think I have an idea why….

The whole criminalization of cannabis thing happened in 1937. America is a lot of things, some good, some pretty crappy, this came from the pretty crappy side.[2] The law was a thinly veiled act of racism used to hurt communities of color, and it worked. In the same way that our federal lawmakers decided that 500g of powdered cocaine was equal to 5g of rock or "crack" (100-to-1 ratio), the criminalization of cannabis was used to prosecute black and brown people in order to keep their communities in check.[3]

As a result, there was a movement that arose in the 60's and 70's, pushing back on those silly laws and sentencing guidelines. It is my belief that many of the individuals making up that movement really did care about change and social justice. The problem we face today comes from that movement being co-opted by people who saw an opportunity to get rich(er). Pretending to care about people, these creative "entrepreneurs" only cared about the money. Using the same language and appearing to care, these people assumed they were a part of a movement, rather than prospectors looking to strike gold. They pulled it off, hijacking arguments around real issues in our nation today and in the past in order to change laws that supported their money-making schemes. That movement has been replaced by an industry, and it's high time we started separating the two when we talk about this issue. The hipsters became hucksters because their feel-good, escape from reality rhetoric and lifestyles didn't put food on the table. They became the new but "enlightened" bourgeoisie, with a work ethic that embraced a ethic of pleasure and self-gratification, replacing the pre-WWII ethic of sacrifice and service. Greed and selfishness have always been part of human DNA, but Americans are good at monetizing it.

The last book was an attempted indictment of this industry and it looks like society is in a place today where they might be more prepared to have this difficult conversation. "Big Weed" is a thing now, something we all accept as real and increasingly "normal." (It's hard to ignore it when you see their stocks scrolling along the bottom of the screen!) A few years ago it felt like there were only a few of us talking about these guys, everyone else was content to assume that it was all mom and pop stuff. It might have started out with a bit of the small time private players but it didn't stay that way for long; the takeover was planned and worked towards from day one. With the tens of billions of dollars being made selling THC these days, I think most of us realize that we have seen the birth of a new industry, a new vice industry.

Not once in the history of this great nation have we done a good job regulating vice substances. Alcohol is by far the most damaging substance in our country; not because it is inherently worse than others but because it is more widely consumed. And it is more widely consumed because there are multibillion dollar corporations dependent on its consumption.[4]

Prescription opiates were around for a long time before we found ourselves in today's "Opioid Crisis." It took those pricks at Purdue Pharma, exploiting the addictive potential of the drugs and gaming the system to their advantage, to get us here today.[5] Then of course there is Big Tobacco. They depend on addiction for profit and their industry kills about 480,000 Americans every year.[6] When capitalism meets addictive substances the results are predictable and problematic.

As I outlined this book and began the halting process of actually writing I had an epiphany: I like writing and dislike research. I get hung up finding and appropriately citing facts, which leads to the enjoyment of the writing process being sucked right out of me. My first inclination was to just write and skip all the stuff nobody reads anyway. Then I realized that just because I don't read the citations in books doesn't mean others are as foolish. As I was considering this problem, fortune struck. I was delivering an address to a group of collegiate athletic professionals alongside my dear friend LaTisha Bader, PhD. When Dr Bader and I finished up, one of the people waiting to talk was a young lady who played Division-1 college golf and was working on an undergrad in some sort of chemistry thing before continuing on for her masters and PhD. She is a high achiever and, as it would turn out, a really cool person. Issy Simpson is her name and she was very interested in the subject and offered to help me research this book. Because it took me so long to write all of this, she has since graduated and moved back to England for her Masters, but she continued to help me along the way. With the aid of a smart, and very patient, researcher I finally felt like I could make a run at writing again.

I've been told that it would have been a bad idea to call this book "I Told You So, Stupid," With that said, "I told ya so." I guess it would be more accurate to say, "We told ya so." Plenty of people have been warning that the weed industry is big tobacco 2.0. Many others warned that we were strengthening the cartels' positions and doing nothing to help the overdose crisis. And I was not alone when we warned that people of color would be locked-up more often and for more time than whites. A host of folks have been talking and writing about these things for a long time.

Let us therefore begin by being perfectly clear; I believe we are moving towards the commercial sales of all drugs and if this takes place it will be done with almost no regulatory oversight or thought given to the innumerable harms and damage it will cause to individual lives and to the fabric of our country. Please don't think small. Think global commercial sales of drugs, because that is the more accurate picture of the broad influence and power that is behind it. What started as "Medical" marijuana became recreational, is now psychedelics and will be opiates and amphetamines. If we continue to believe all that is being told to us by those selling marijuana and other substances and refuse to question their motives and integrity, it will be our own fault when we find ourselves with commercial sales of even more drugs; led by those who need addiction to drive profits and do not care about the damage they cause. The stakes are very high right now and it is past time that we apply critical thought to this issue.

That is the last that I'm going to mention the "other drugs' ' thing, at least for a bit. The last thing we need is for the reader to assume that I wear a tinfoil cap to bed, so let's get back to weed. First thing's first, <u>we need to stop calling it "weed."</u>

Unless you have purchased and consumed a marijuana based product intended to intoxicate from a commercial establishment/dispensary (not the CBD oil on Amazon or your hemp soap from Whole Foods) in the last year or two, you don't know about today's "weed". You are operating under a construct about marijuana that is so antiquated it is irrelevant at best. I say "at best" because ignorance of something can lead one to ignore or even enable something that should not be ignored or encouraged all the while thinking we know what we're doing. For example, remember how long it took us to believe that we might not know all we thought we knew about cigarette smoke, or trans-fat, asbestos, global warming or Harvey Weinstein? We thought we knew, but in hindsight we didn't and it probably would have been good to understand sooner.

What I want to do right now is to challenge us to change our language when talking about "weed". We do a huge disservice to this conversation by limiting and muddling our vocabulary, using a few words to discuss an extremely diverse line of products and variations, we are no longer just deciding between the two main 'types' of cannabis, indica and sativa, the world has radically changed since the industrialization of marijuana.

We use word(s) like "weed," "cannabis," "marijuana," or "sticky-icky" pretty loosely, oftentimes without even knowing what it is we are referencing. "Weed" has changed so much in the last few years that saying "marijuana" is kinda like saying "liquid." There's a big difference between orange juice and whisky, between hot cocoa and kale juice, gasoline and Sprite. Get the picture? To make the point more clearly, imagine trying to communicate about liquid with only one word to distinguish what we were talking about:

"Dude, can you speak a bit more softly, I had like 18 cans of liquid last night."

"I understand you aren't feeling well, I want you to take two teaspoons of liquid and call me in the morning"

"Mmmmmm, I think I'd like a glass of liquid with my steak please."

"Don't forget to pick up some liquid at the store, honey."

Unclear and maybe even unsafe, right? It's the same thing with weed. For example, I remember when CNN's Dr. Sanjay Gupta declared that "weed stops seizures." He made a big statement that was more inaccurate than accurate.[7] A more accurate declaration would have been something like this: "The non-intoxicating component of the cannabis plant, called CBD, manufactured by the Stanley Brothers into a serum called 'Charlotte's Web' shows promise treating a rare seizure disorder called Devrot Syndrome in several patients I met." While a statement like this would have been much more accurate, it wouldn't have driven viewership to CNN, or get hits on YouTube or retweets. So, the headlines it generated and Gupta's quote "...Would not just be a medical failing but a moral failing if this medicine was somehow withheld from people" reads in a much more general and simpler yet confusing way. It's time we started talking about "weed" in a more informed way; not confusing medicine with concentrated marijuana, differentiating between a plant that is smoked and an extract that is eaten, between an herb and a topical cream.

In 2023 "weed" can be smoked, eaten, absorbed topically, inhaled, vaped, inserted into one's anus or vagina, drank, chewed, turned into paper and shoes and dropped into one's eyes. It has taken on a diversity like "liquid," yet our vernacular has not kept up. Allow me to expand your understanding and vocabulary.......

Marijuana is a plant, often referred to as cannabis in scientific and some political circles. It's a plant that we have interacted with for thousands of years. It grows in warm places, consumes large amounts of water and, when dried and smoked, can have a subtly intoxicating effect; especially the un-pollinated buds of the female plant. In 2012, my home state of Colorado redefined marijuana when we passed the constitutional amendment #64. Since then every state to pass "recreational" marijuana laws has followed suit, by legally, yet inaccurately, defining marijuana as follows:

"MARIJUANA" OR "MARIHUANA" MEANS ALL PARTS OF THE PLANT OF THE GENUS CANNABIS WHETHER GROWING OR NOT, THE SEEDS THEREOF, THE RESIN EXTRACTED FROM ANY PART OF THE PLANT, AND EVERY COMPOUND, MANUFACTURE, SALT, DERIVATIVE, MIXTURE, OR PREPARATION OF THE PLANT, ITS SEEDS, OR ITS RESIN, INCLUDING MARIHUANA CONCENTRATE...."[8]

The voters of Colorado, somewhat unknowingly, changed the traditional definition of weed when we agreed to the language in A64 and many have followed suit. Since the new and legal way of defining "weed" has replaced the long-standing traditional meaning, I hope you get curious about terms like "concentrates" and "resin" "Compounds, Manufacture, Salt, Derivatives and Mixtures." The new, legal definition means we can use the entire plant, change its form and consume it in uncountable ways that would never fit under the traditional and scientific definition.

I'm going to give you some new words and attempt to describe them. I'm also throwing in a few pics, because guys like me need pictures and because some of this stuff is hard to imagine. As always, you can probably learn just as much by a quick Google search (make sure to run "image" searches) or by spending a little bit of time on YouTube. If you want to see what it looks like to consume any of what follows I can pretty much guarantee that there are dozens of YouTube channels dedicated to it.

Marijuana

Let's start with an easy one. Marijuana is "weed." "Weed" is marijuana. "Cannabis" is the scientific name. It's a naturally-occurring plant, growing in warm environments and requiring large amounts of water to grow. In its natural form it contains less than .5% THC, that is the part of the plant that gets you high.[9] Humankind has always interacted with this natural plant. We didn't really smoke it until recently, and we used it for several of its medicinal properties. We have also used it as a cash crop, commonly referred to as "hemp"; more on that later.[10] Not too long ago we started to mess with the genetics of the plant in order to get it to grow better in colder climates and, of course, to get us high. At some point somebody figured out that by increasing the THC, by means of rudimentary botany, it had a bit of a relaxing and even subtle intoxicating effect. Since some people like to get intoxicated, a few people got really into using, and eventually smoking, cannabis in order to get kinda, sorta, a little bit stoned.

In the early 70's we started to see a consistent increase in the amount of THC being bred into weed. It went gangbusters, relatively speaking, between when Led Zeppelin was smoking it and when Snoop Dog hit the scene in the early 90's. By the time Miley Cyrus picked it up, THC had grown to an incredible average of approximately 12% THC nationwide.[11] In just forty-some years, marijuana potency had grown by a multiplier of 20-ish!

A while back, I was giving a talk and a young man asked me if I thought that marijuana had influenced music in a positive way. After getting a good laugh at the creativity of the question, I told him that I thought it likely had. Plenty of the artists, whose music we now consider as "classics," consumed their fair share of yesterday's weed. Personally, I think the world is a better place because of "Purple Haze" and the works of Pink Floyd, not to mention the activist genius of Bob Marley. All of those fellas, I believe, enjoyed their weed. But, the weed consumed back then was a more natural form of marijuana (low THC).

That's not to say their creativity was a result of marijuana intoxication, but substance use can usually offer a desirable effect of a change in perspective, or the permission to engage in a creative activity long after the unaltered mind has moved on to other tasks. This has been the experience of creative thinkers, innovators and others with out-of-the-box perspectives since the beginning of time. But a note of caution, we can also conjure up a list of creative spirits that didn't survive the process of creating when substances were added to their process.

Hemp

There was an old saying, "The most dangerous thing about weed is getting caught with it."   At one time that was pretty darn true. When we first criminalized weed, we were really criminalizing hemp. Sadly, we did it back then so the fellas in charge could make more money on their textiles as well as find ways to put more black and brown people in jail. In the 2018 Farm Bill, "hemp" was legally defined as having less than .3% THC. That means, today's Hemp was yesterday's weed![12]

Hemp has lots of uses. (I'm not really an expert on them, ask a farmer.) What I know is that it's used as a tough and lightweight textile for a wide variety of products, including my favorite pair of shoes.

The trick with hemp, and the reason that my buddies in law enforcement aren't big fans of it, is that it looks VERY similar to weed. That allows the outlaws to grow it in the perfect camo, a field bordered by hemp. Unfortunately, for the people whose job it is to keep weed out of the black market, hemp makes their task much harder.

CBD

This is the part of the cannabis plant with the medicine in it. It is super important to understand that <u>CBD is totally nonintoxicating</u>, like totally. According to your nephew, or anyone who's been brainwashed by popular marketing, CBD will fix everything from cancer to global warming. Many believe we should basically get as much as we can into and on our bodies as often as possible. While a good deal of the benefits to CBD are simply anecdotal, it does have some scientifically- validated medical benefits. I wouldn't be surprised that as we study it further we find a few more. We know that CBD is an anti-inflammatory and a pretty remarkable anti-convulsant.[13,14] What we don't know about CBD is how it interacts with other medications, its long-term effects, proper dose and concentrations, or the most effective delivery systems.

For all of the good and potential good that we know and are learning about CBD, today's market has one giant problem; nobody really agrees on a single definition of CBD. Scientifically we know exactly what it is, how to isolate it, how to measure it, and even how to synthesize it. But practically, anything can be labeled CBD because there is no federal oversight of this booming marketplace, allowing anybody to sell anything and claim it is CBD. I have seen creams bought off the shelf at a grocery store and repackaged as "CBD". There are people passing off liquids/edibles/oils/capsules or whatever else that contain trace amounts of CBD as "CBD based" products. The marketplace lacks a universally-accepted definition of what actually constitutes a product as "CBD based." The absence of a clear definition allows for just about anything to be passed off as CBD. As you might imagine, this is a problem for a multitude of reasons. Consider these examples.

At one point in 2020, a product search of Bed Bath and Beyond offered 68 different products claiming to contain CBD, ranging from lip balm, to bracelets and to pillow cases. Prices ranged from $150 to $19.99. A local hardware store was the purveyor of a CBD infused fire log; three for $35. During a walk in City Park, I discovered you could enjoy a CBD infused hot dog for $10. A well-known saying is one of my favorites: "Buyer beware."

Medical Marijuana

This is a tough one, which will probably frustrate lots of people. Sorry, but we have to define what this is. I believe a medicine can be defined as "a product that has been validated to have measurable and repeatable specific effects on specific conditions by double blind, placebo controlled testing". Additionally, a medicine comes with a dosage amount and a duration of effectiveness. Almost never is a true medicine used as much as one desires until one feels what one desires to feel. And to be perfectly clear, there isn't a medicine on earth that is smoked. Let me say it again, "You don't smoke medicine, ever!" Using the definition above, there are four forms of "Medical Marijuana," or more accurately, "cannabis derived medications": Dronabinol & Nabilone (which contain some THC) and Epidiolex & Sativex (which contain no THC).[15,16]

In order to try a shift in perspective, say the phrase "I can't wait to take my Jack Daniels medication." We know alcohol can provide a biphasic response (first 1-2 drinks is euphoric, after that it's a depressant). For some, this can be a very desirable experience, but that doesn't make Jack Daniels a true medicine.

Also, consider the emotional connection we have with medications. I can't think of one morning when I awoke and had the thought, "I can't wait to get my dose of fish oil." Medications aren't often mind/mood altering. For that reason, we don't often develop a psychological bond to them. We appreciate that they treat our symptoms or provide prevention, and that's usually where our connection with medicine stops. When medications can and do alter our mind and mood, we exert great caution with prescribing and using them, because of addictive potential, physical and emotional.

It is dangerous when something can be dubbed "medicine" by popular vote. We should stay far away from that kind of standard. One key reason, and one I believe is most relevant, is that medicines have known side-effects. Think of the commercials for medications that run on TV; they are compelled to list the potential harms associated with that medication, some of which sound way worse than what the medication treats. When we introduce powerful substances into our brains and bodies there will be side effects. Currently, "Medical Marijuana" is being discussed without this important consideration. What we hear are nothing but success stories with little or no discussion of the harms, of which there are plenty. This is irresponsible. Imagine if the pharma companies producing medications weren't compelled to tell us the potential harms, do you think they would? We allow medical marijuana to be defined by the companies and industry groups profiting on them. They tell us nothing but the good, ignoring or downplaying the negative. We are setting ourselves up for trouble because people, some of them very sick and dying, aren't given the whole story, just the parts that sell.

It is past time that we not only separate "medical" from "recreational" when discussing marijuana but that we get serious about advancing research into the real medical properties of the plant.

To clarify what's going on, I would like to ask this question, "What is the difference between "medical" and recreational marijuana?" The answer is, "Nothing!" The only differences are cost (taxes) and age of access (18 vs 21). But if one is "medical," these questions must be addressed and spelled out: how does one use it; when does one use it;, and why does one use it?

Marijuana Concentrate

While most people don't have any idea what a "concentrate" is, they have quickly become a major, if not predominant, part of the commercial market. For example, the last year that we have full sales data out of Colorado is 2020. That year we taxed the sale of just over 42,000 pounds of "concentrated marijuana". While that might not seem like a lot, please understand that the manufacturers encourage users to consume an amount "half the size of a pinhead or less."

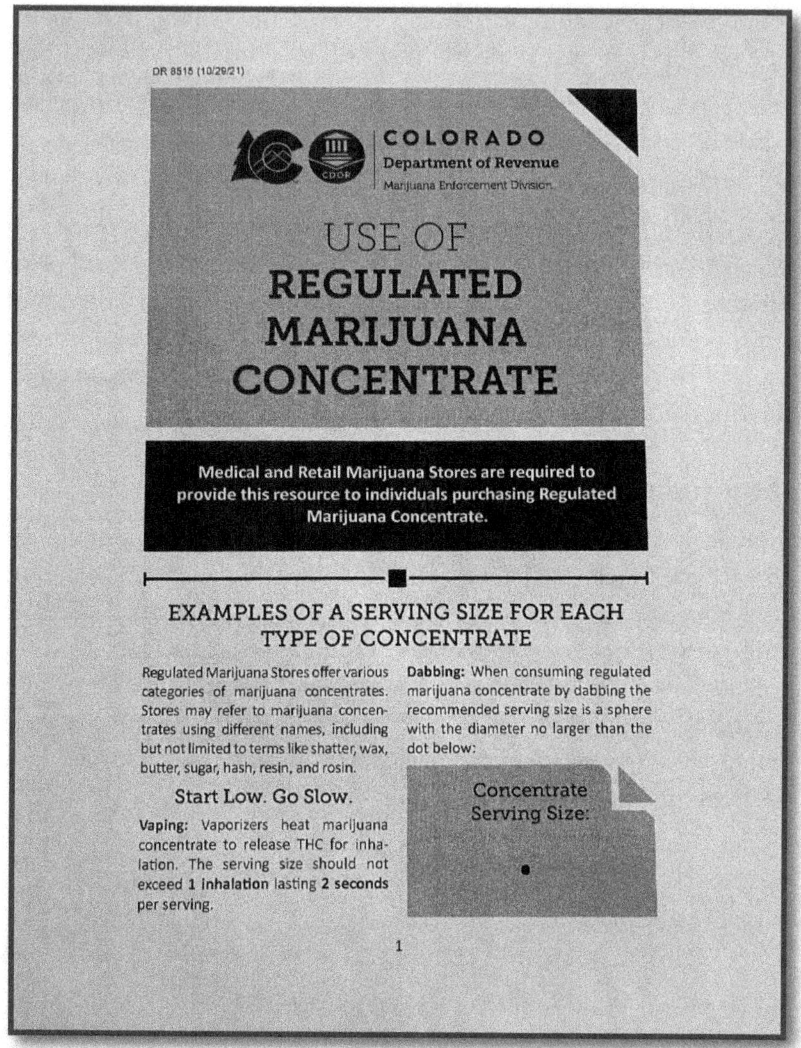

Colorado's Marijuana Enforcement Division calculated that the legal market sold over 11.5 million servings of concentrates in 2020.[17] The industry claims that people will moderate their use because it is so strong, but this misses the well-documented reality of tolerance to THC. A quick YouTube search will show as many people as you want to watch consuming amounts in excess of 5 grams of THC in one sitting.

Defining a concentrate is pretty easy; it's THC stripped from the organic plant material. This is most commonly done with a solvent, such as butane or propane, that "grabs" the THC. Depending on how it is made, THC can also be separated out with gravity, compression, cold water, etc.[18] Concentrates can take lots of forms and contain 40-99% THC.[19] Now is a good time to remember the earlier definition of marijuana. In case you forgot, the plant in its natural form should contain less than .5% THC. Since the potency of concentrated THC is so new, the scientific/ medical community knows next to nothing about how THC levels this extreme are affecting the brain and body. I can tell you some stories, based on my years of watching from the front row, and say pretty confidently that they are not doing much good. There is a growing body of evidence telling us of the risks of psychosis associated with higher potency, above 10% THC.[20] Since the science regarding concentrates is relevant to both individuals and to society, it needs to be weighed carefully.

The problem is made much worse because concentrates are worth lots more than the naturally-occuring marijuana plant. Concentrates are easy to make and result in much higher use rates. For these reasons, the marijuana industry loves them. Asking the industry to give up their concentrates is like trying to get my 13-year-old to eat broccoli, it just isn't happening. The concentrate industry will go to the mat in order to keep this valuable and ever growing piece of their market in stores.

While we have defined marijuana concentrates as a whole, I think it is important to understand the specific forms they have taken in today's marketplace. (I'm guessing that this list will be outdated by the time you read it but we've got to start somewhere!) Commonly used names and local advertisements are listed below.

Wax

This is the stuff made from butane. It is less pure and in its final form looks like beeswax.[21]

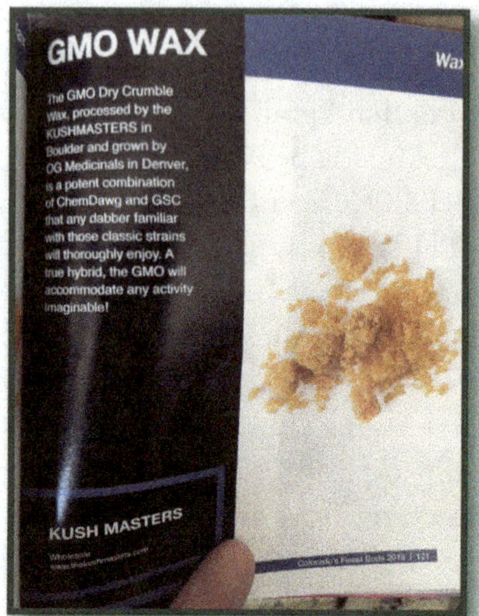

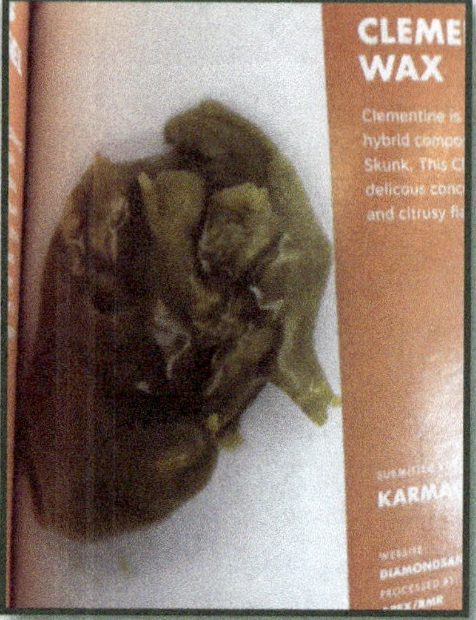

Shatter

Made from multiple filtrations of leftover resin, resulting in a thin, glass sheet, that is easily "shattered."[22]

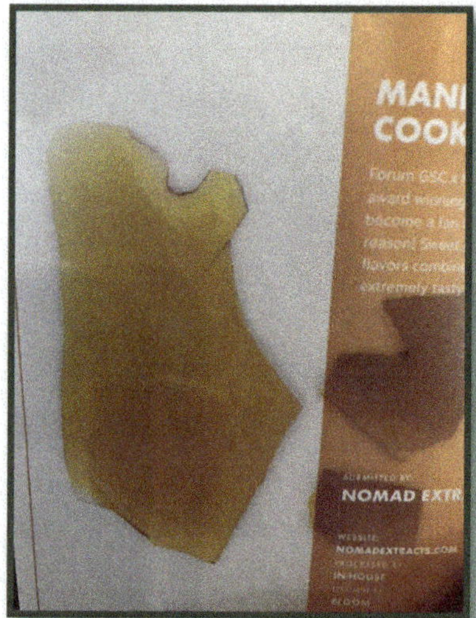

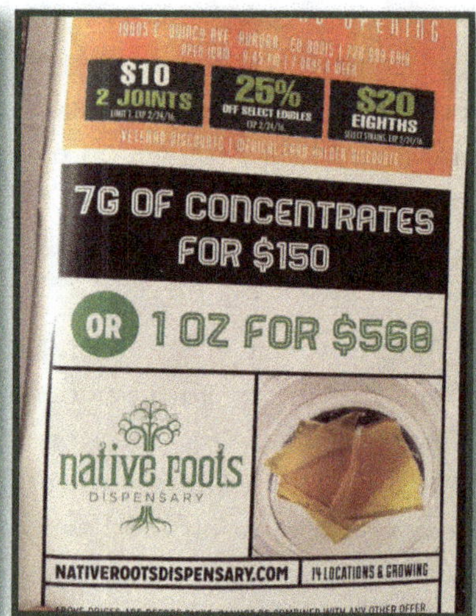

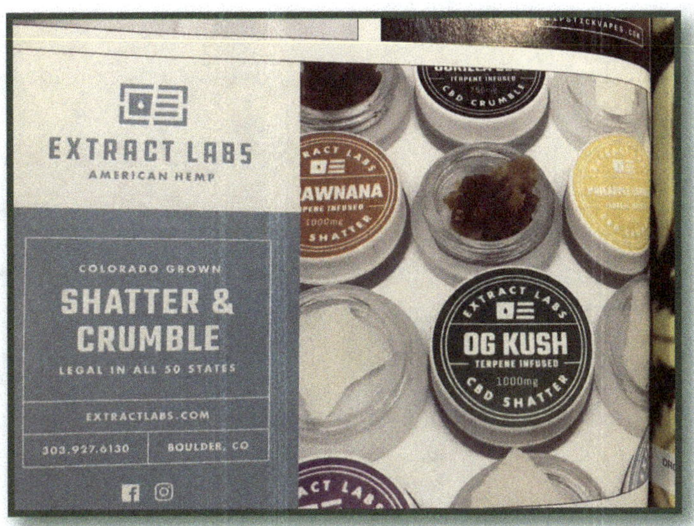

Sauce

Derived from a flash frozen, whole plant, it preserves more than just the THC. In Sauce, the plant properties that produce specific smells and tastes (called "terpenes"), are also extracted.[23]

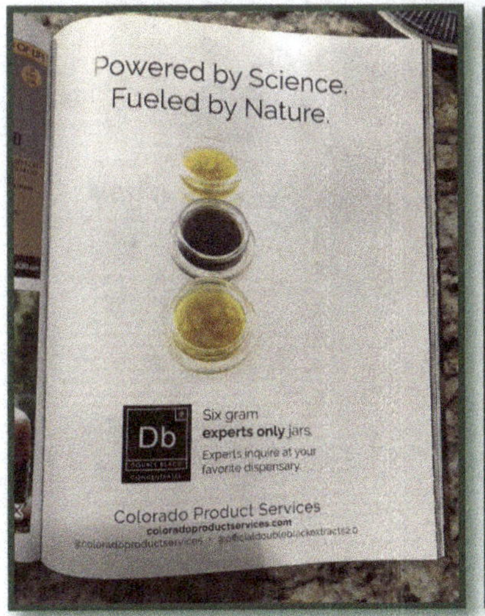

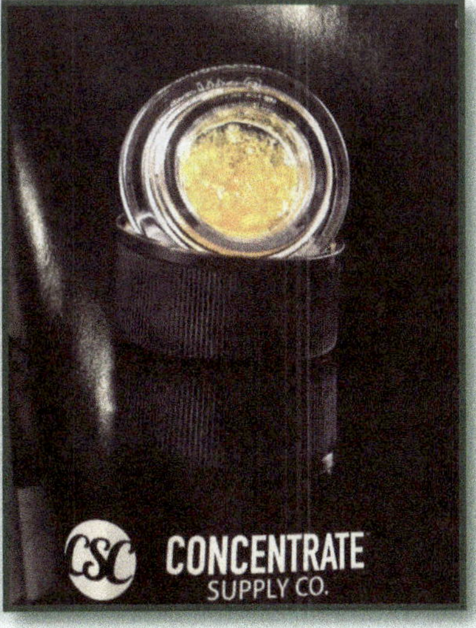

Live Resin

This product is also flash frozen. Typically it is considered to have more flavor[24]

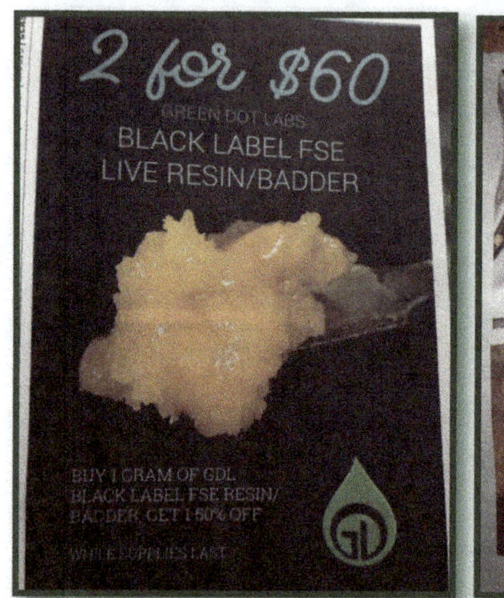

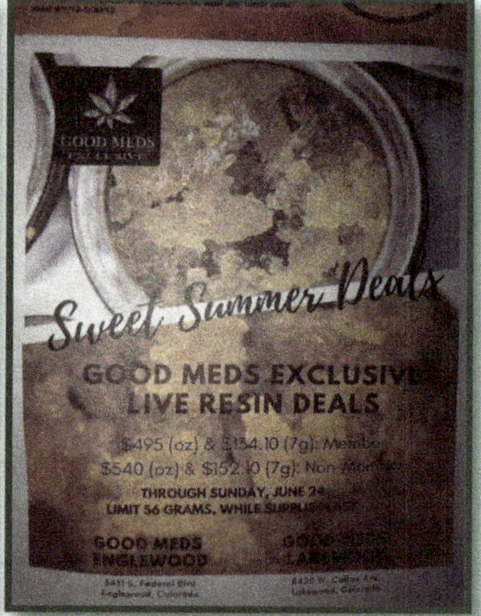

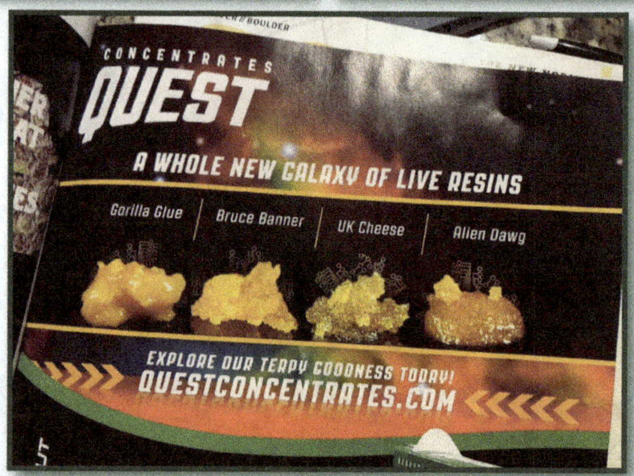

Solventless

Rather than using things like butane and CO_2, this product is produced by using techniques like gravity and cold water reverse osmosis to extract THC.[25]

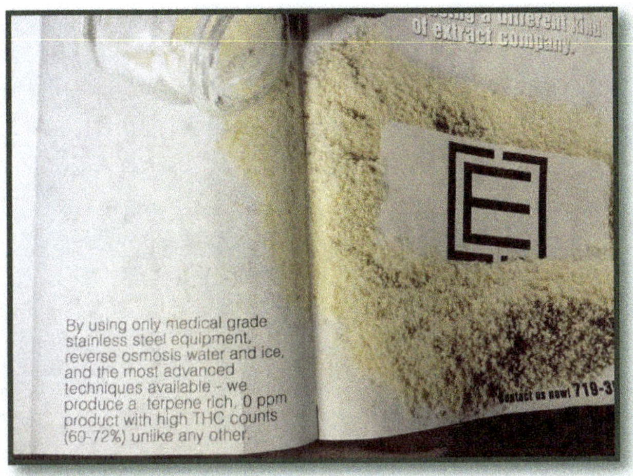

Distillates

I think these very new and popular products will become the future of the cannabis industry to some degree. At most marijuana dispensaries they are front and center and are fast becoming a favorite to vape and infuse into edibles. Distillates are THC isolated at the molecular level to allow the most pure form of THC, the delta-9 (the most potent part of THC), to be consumed on its own. It is basically the world's first pure form of non-synthesized THC. Its potency tests as high as 99.9% THC.[26]

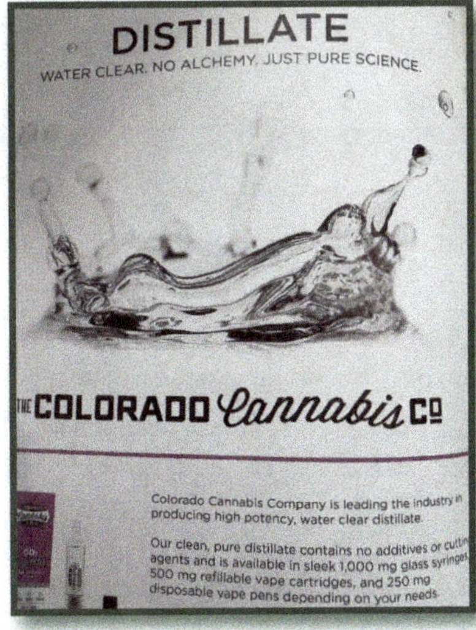

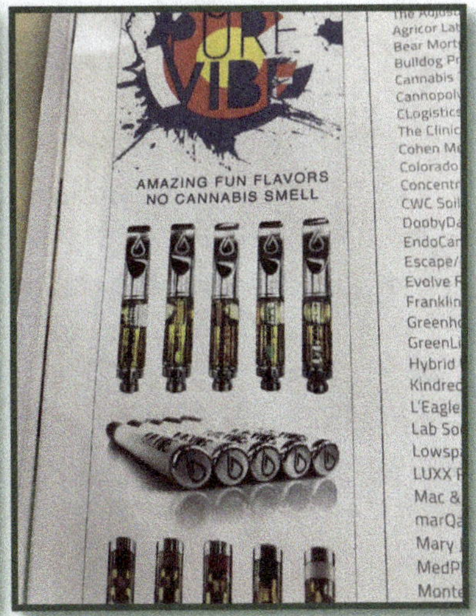

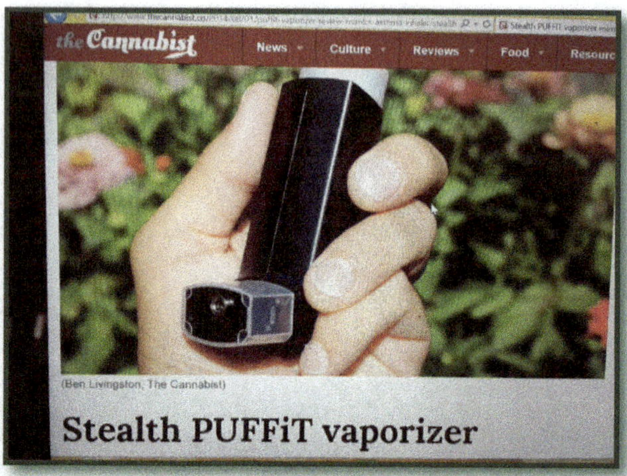

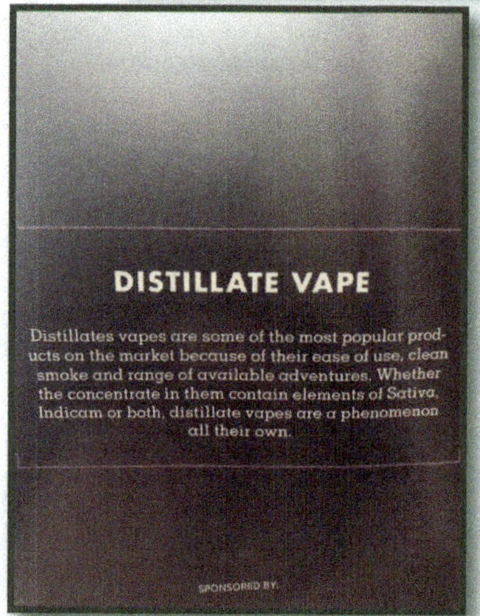

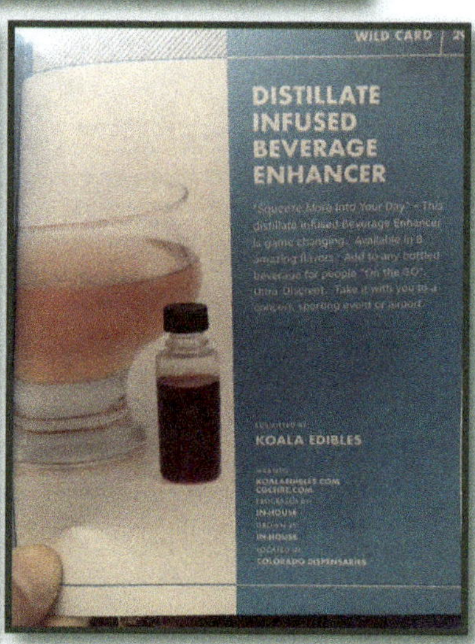

Given the large variation in the potency of concentrates, it's important to understand a few of the more popular forms in which they are marketed. Since something with the consistency of a jolly rancher can't be rolled up and smoked like a traditional "joint," look for these to be consumed in vaporizers, smoked on a super heated needle or in a glass pipe. If you are aware of other illicit drugs that are consumed in rock form, you will understand how these are smoked.

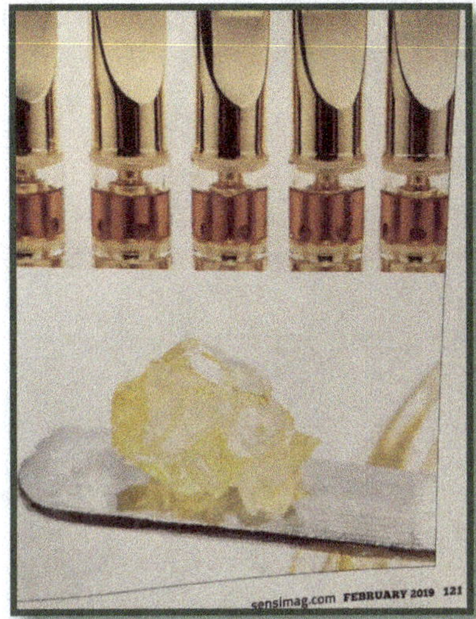

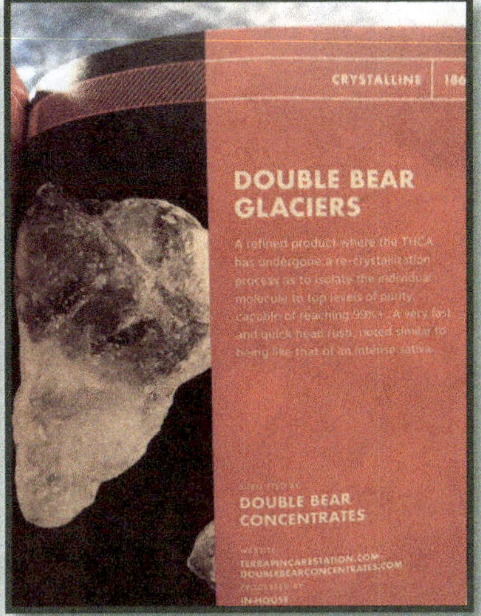

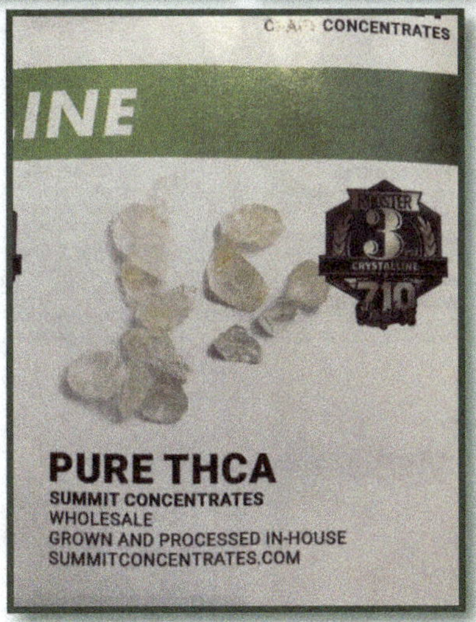

Edibles

We have entered an era in which anything that can be introduced into the human body is being produced with THC, often concentrated THC. If you are like me, you think of an edible as a baked good, like a brownie or cookie. This understanding is extremely antiquated when it comes to THC because these consumables now cover an extremely diverse and wide range of commercial products. For example, THC is infused in…

Water, juice, lemonade, tea, coffee, honey, beer, soda, gummies, hard candies, soft candies, fudge, chocolates, ice cream, condiments, pills, suckers, gum, mints, breath spray, toothpicks, candy bars, peanut butter cups, gum, potato chips, syrup, and butter (allowing it to be cooked into anything)!

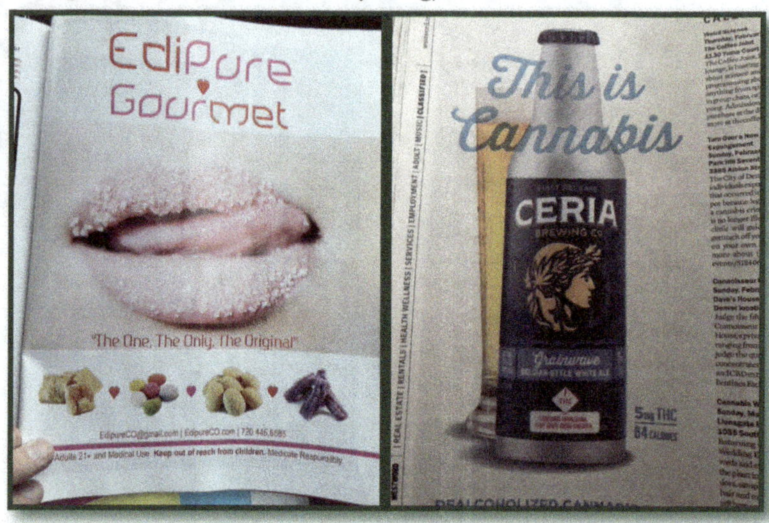

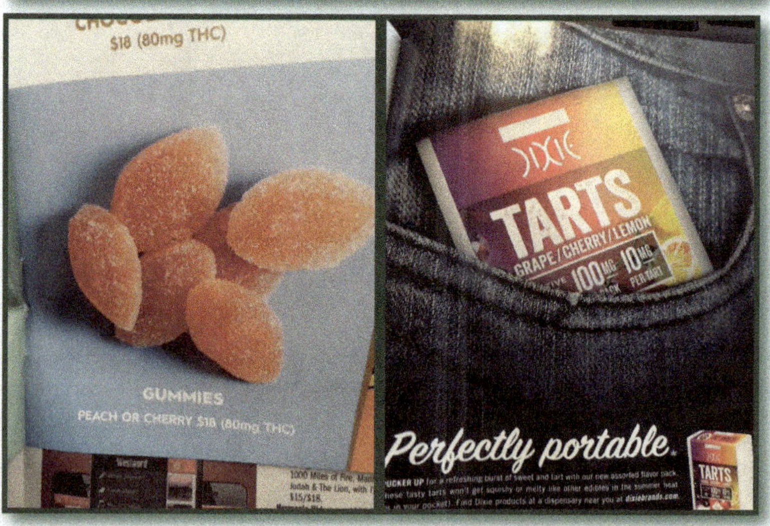

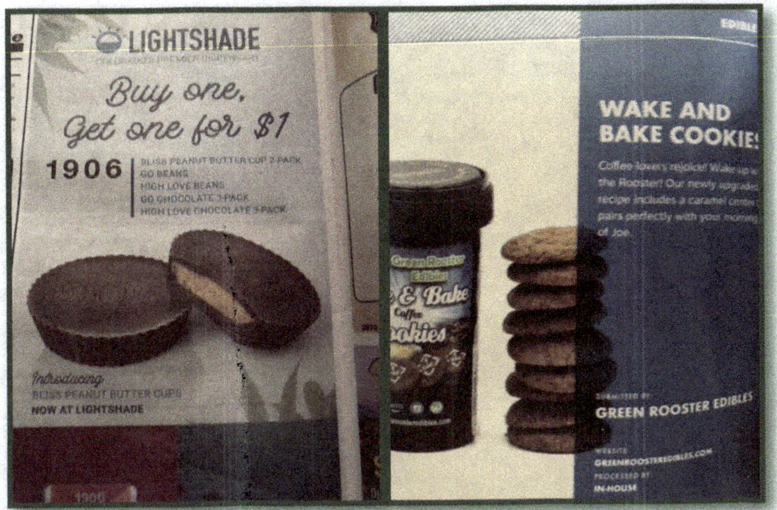

CBD makes its way into our bodies through the same "routes of administration" and often with much higher doses, think hundreds of mg!

In terms of science and the body, "routes of administration" incorporate the stomach, liver and digestive track. In the first pass through the metabolism, the liver identifies the THC as a foreign substance and processes it as toxin. It begins to break it down into 11-hydrox-THC, which is now more potent than the original THC that the person consumed. So, the original concentration is now more concentrated! Metabolism of THC and 11-hydrox-THC is long lasting, increasing the high.[27]

For this reason, it is imperative that THC-infused edibles be regulated. Even WIllie Nelson has sworn off edibles because of a bad trip. That should be enough inspiration!

Topicals

These include intoxicating creams, nasal sprays, eye drops, intimate oils, and even suppositories!

Okay, there ya have it; you are an expert on all things weed! Now that you know, it is your responsibility to use this knowledge, change your vocabulary and help those around you to change theirs. This should also help a great deal while reading what follows.

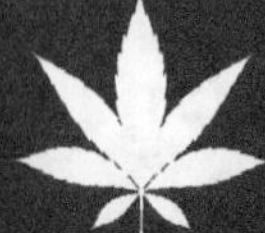

CHAPTER

02

THE RICH GET RICHER

But They Still Want More

The Aug/Sept issue of Forbes magazine has the CEO of a cannabis company on the cover. Gilbert Anthony Milam Jr., AKA "Berner", whose net worth is listed as $20m is the first, and I am guessing not the last, cannabis industry executive to grace the cover of the nation's foremost magazine about wealth and industry. In many ways Gilbert is an enigma; he is a minority and did not attend an ivy league school like most of his peers in the industry. On 8/4/22, the daily newsletter from MJbizdaily hit my inbox. I opened it up to see what the latest news was in the industry. The headline read, "Seven US marijuana CEO's saw compensation top $4m in 2021".[1] The list of millionaires includes, not surprisingly, an all male cast with one female. Here is the list with their cash and stock earnings for 2021:

1. George Archos (Loyola University)
   Verano Holdings
   $16.03m

2. Abner Kurtin (Horace Mann and Harvard MBA)
   Ascend Wellness
   $15.96m

3. James Cacioppo (Colgate University, Harvard MBA)
   Jushi Holdings
   $9.87m

4. Kim Rivers (Florida State and University of Florida)
   Trulieve Cannabis
   $8.05m

5. Robert Groesbeck (University of Nevada, National University, Western Michigan)
   Planet 13 Holdings
   $6.5m

6. Larry Scheffler (unsure of education but he became a lawyer in there somewhere)
   Planet 13 Holdings
   $6.49m

The same article goes on to tell us that of the top fifteen paid executives in the industry, Kim Rivers is the only female, the rest are white men. One of those men is a Columbia Care (a big ol' weed company) co-founder. CEO Nicholas Vita whose total compensation for the year could exceed $100m following an acquisition.

Since this is a chapter exposing nepotism and underhanded dealings, I would like to share a bit more about Kim. While many would like to celebrate the only female in that group for making the list and pushing the ceiling, I propose that rather than changing anything she has just joined the rich boys club. In November 2021 Kim's husband, J.T. Burnette, was sentenced to 3 years in prison and a fine of $1.25m in Florida for a bribery scheme. To be more specific, he was found guilty of one count of extortion, two counts of honest service fraud by bribery, and one count of use of interstate commerce facilities to promote bribery. Back in 2016, when Kim and J.T. were still dating, he was recorded by an undercover FBI agent bragging about how he used political connections to tweek the new medical marijuana (MMJ) in order to make sure that Kim's company got a license and her competitors did not.

Kim and her company wrote a very lovely letter of support asking for leniency when J.T. was sentenced, one might expect this from a loving and supportive wife. Kim was also clearly motivated by their business relationship as much as their personal one. It turns out that she had awarded J.T.'s company, 'Burnette Construction,' over $230m in construction projects for her weed company.

Recently, I was giving a virtual talk to a group of professionals in Georgia. In the opening comments, the gentleman setting the stage was talking about GA going from a "medical" state to a recreational state. He played a local news clip featuring Kim in which she shared what appeared to be a very heartfelt message about how this was just about the suffering patients. There are plenty of "carpetbagger" quotes from her interviews in GA after they got the first license, but my favorite is "I look forward to improving the lives of Geogians with much needed and long-awaited medicine."[2] Is it really about the patients? In her home state of Florida, even with EXCEPTIONALLY liberal qualifying conditions, there are only a potential 844,000 qualified patients (4 percent of the population there), whereas over two times that number use recreationally.[3] So for the company to really grow, recreational must be the end game because for every potential medical user there are two already using recreational users.

This section had to be amended before publishing because of some nutty stuff that happened over at Trulive Cannabis. Turns out the company, run by the only female in the crew mentioned above, has been in trouble for their discriminatory hiring, pay and promotion! In April 2023, they settled a suit from an African-American female employee, named Brooke Bennett. Ms. Bennett's suit called out the company for paying entry level black workers $.50 less than white workers, as well as for racial and gender discrimination, retaliation, and for receiving lower compensation than white colleagues in the same position.[4] In addition to Ms. Bennett's now settled suit, as of this writing seven similar suits remain open for Trulive.

Despite all of this, Trulieve and their shiny white senior leadership team, as well as their white-as-snow board of directors, managed to get an award for "Corporate Diversity"! The group that gave it to them, Minorities for Medical Marijuana, is a nonprofit based in Winter Garden, FL. I was curious how an organization with a solid history of discriminatory practices could get this award. Although nonprofits have to file something called a "990" with the IRS so the world can see how they get and spend their money, it appears Minorities for Medical Marijuana haven't filed taxes since 2017.

In addition to racist practices, Trulive landed in hot water last year when on Juneteenth they ran a special on Banana Kush and Grape and Watermelon strains of their weed.[5] For those unfamiliar with discriminatory jargon and stereotypes, banana, grape and watermelon have deeply racist undertones directed at the black community. When Twitter lit them up, Kim's company got all defensive and then all apologetic; demonstrating the disingenuous corporate American "mia culpa"! Their Twitter post said in part "….in light of the culturally insensitive promotional lineup sent earlier today…." Say whatever you want Trulive but if it walks like a duck, quacks like a duck, looks like a duck and a bunch of the people who work there are saying "yo it's a duck" maybe it is!

Well, enough about Kim. I don't know her, but I'm appalled at her hypocrisy and greed. And as far as her hubby goes, he is a perfect example of what is wrong with this country. No matter how much he has he needs more, and he believes rules don't apply to him. Nothing is off limits so long as you get a bigger boat. Well, I hope he makes some friends in prison who help him understand that he is not exceptional.

Ganjaprenuer is one of my favorite news sources reporting in the THC industry. Their daily email contains headlines that do a better job breaking down the widespread commercialization and money-grabbing in the THC market than I could ever do. A recent email said that Steve DeAngelo had penned an op-ed that was "making waves" in the industry. The article, entitled "Save the Cannabis Industry, Topple the Pyramids," described how big corporate interests and investment bankers, "newcomers with mainstream business backgrounds," had "set up massive cultivation centers, developed their planting plans more according to spreadsheets than deep experience or love of the plant".[6]

Those of you who are new to this conversation may be asking "who is Steve DeAngelo"? Steve is "father of the legal cannabis industry," according to the former mayor of San Francisco, Willie L. Brown. Here is an excerpt from Steve's website bio: 'Steve DeAngelo is a pioneering cannabis entrepreneur, activist, author, and on-screen personality. He co-founded several iconic cannabis businesses and organizations: Harborside, one of the first six dispensaries licensed in the US; Steep Hill Laboratory, the first dedicated cannabis lab; the Arc View Group, the first cannabis investment firm; and the National Cannabis Industry Association, the industry's first trade association."[7] Here is the perfect example of what happens when the dog catches the car.

For decades Steve chased the car of commercial sales, telling us all how much better things would be if we just let it happen. In a tweet from 9/5/22, Steve writes, "In the last five years we've seen many examples of how NOT to legalize cannabis."[8] Steve was ticked-off and I suggest that much of his attitude comes from a loss of market share more than a love of the plant. I have no doubt that Steve started out in this for many of the right reasons. He spends a good deal of time bringing awareness to people who are locked up for silly weed related crimes and seems to care a great deal for disenfranchised communities. However the fourth paragraph of his recent op-ed may shed light into additional motivations driving Steve's business ventures. Here it is in its entirety (emphasis mine):

'Everything changed on January 1, 2018. The day before, Harborside had been supplied by over 500 small, independent cannabis farmers. The day after, we discovered that only 10 of those growers had been able to secure state licenses. At the same time, out on the sales floor, our prices increased by 40% because of ridiculous tax schemes enacted by all levels of government— city, county, and state. So **consumers ran out of our doors with sticker shock, right into the arms of all the growers who had not been licensed. We immediately began to see a drop in sales, for the first time in our history**— and the same thing happened to licensed dispensaries across the state."[9]

Could it be that the author of the "cannabis manifesto" is really driven, at least in part, by simple profit? In a 12/3/21 article on Benzinga, entitled "Meet 9 of the richest people in the cannabis industry," and then republished on "Fresh Toast" by the same author to include the "10 richest people in the cannabis industry," Steve DeAngelo is listed as #8, just ahead of Snoop Dog. Much of his immense wealth is because of his role co-found-ing ArcView Group, a cannabis investment firm with over 600 investors controlling about $200m, not to mention the declared earnings from Harborside (Steve's company) that top $35m.[10] So, Steve is not only living in the lap of luxury, but he has a fiduciary duty to return as much as possible to his investors. Yet, he is apparently edged out by even bigger players, like #'s 1-7, which is topped by Brandon Kennedy.

Brandon Kennedy is co-founder of a rival investment group called "Privateer Holdings," which at one time was worth over $2b but has been recently reduced following a stock crash to a mere $200m personal net worth. Privateer Holdings controls about $228m in capital. On January 6, 2019, Fortune Magazine featured Kennedy in an article called "The Marijuana Billionaire Who Doesn't Smoke Weed". The article's tagline is revealing: "With the help of Big Beer and Big Pharma, Brendan Kennedy's Canadian cannabis company Tilray has unexpectedly become America's gateway to the legal marijuana industry." Jeff Lewis, the first guy to invest big money with Kennedy, is quoted in the article as saying, "The first entrepreneur who didn't offer him a taste? Brendan Kennedy. And that's what I wanted to invest in—I wanted a team that didn't use cannabis."[11] Jeff is a smart guy, he wanted businessmen not consumers or advocates. Kennedy and his crew do not use THC, they know better. It's reminiscent of the executive at R.J. Reynolds who famously said "We don't smoke this shit, we just sell it. We reserve the right to smoke for the young, the poor, the Black, and the stupid."[12]

Make no mistake, these are different people but motivated by the same greed and disregard for others, other than themselves. The guys who were big tobacco, big pharma, and big alcohol (the most damaging substance on earth) are the guys running the big cannabis firms. Take David Klein for example, the CEO of Canopy Growth which is the largest cannabis firm in the world.

David joined Canopy in 2020 after 16 years at Constellation Brands, one of the largest owners of alcohol brands in the world. Prior to becoming CEO, David was on the board for two years.

Canopy knew that they needed the know-how of the alcohol industry and David was perfect for the job. Apparently, he is not an exception. The University of Bath has done a nice job cataloging some of the crossover between tactics from tobacco to cannabis and from senior executives and scientists leaving tobacco to get in on the green rush. Check out their page called "Tobacco Tactics" to learn more.[13] On 9/27/22, High Times magazine ran an article "Is Big Tobacco Pivoting To Big Cannabis." It pointed out that Philip Morris is owned by a company called Altria, which owns "altriacannabis.com."[14]

Next, let's look at the powerful and profitable pharmaceutical companies, "Pharma." There has not been a more devastating product than OxyContin in recent history. It killed and kills lots of people every year. One of the senior executives from Purdue Pharma (Jonathan Stewart), one of the key players behind the opiate crisis, left that company in 2013 to found Emblem Cannabis. It is a Canadian company that literally says on it's website "Become a patient. Easy as 1-2-3. Ready to try medical cannabis but worried about a lengthy application process? Becoming an Emblem Cannabis patient is surprisingly easy." It sells products like "bogarts kitchen soft mango chews," "limited edition powdered doughnuts bud," "Divy Pineapple" pre rolled Joints, and 12 flavors of THC vape cartridges.[15] I think there is a special place in hell for all of those Purdue guys and it looks like this one is trying his best to be the worst. He took everything he learned about addicting 'patients' to opiates and is applying it to THC.

While I considered wrapping this chapter up here, with the tobacco, alcohol and oxy guys, I just can't, there are too many other people to call out. Let's talk about celebrities!

For the most part, just about all of the examples I can find of minorities making money in the cannabis industry are people who came into it with great wealth and used that wealth and name recognition to pile money on top of money. The idea of social equity inside the world of weed is laughable. Even as states try to pass laws so minorities can get in on the riches the money always

45

ends up with the rich white guys, or as listed below the rich and famous minorities. Here are a few ethnic minorities who are killing it in legal weed with their own brands and ventures:*

- Snoop Dogg ("bitches ain't shit but ho's and tricks…" he said that but I'm sure he would love it if you ladies bought his concentrate THC)

- Jay Z ($1.3b net worth before the weed thing)

- The Marley Estate (Bob was a religious man and an activist, he is rolling over in his grave as his image and legacy are being used to get and keep people high rather than fight for awareness and social justice)

- Wiz Khalifa (I don't know much about these kids today. He is super rich, has lots of tattoos and loves THC.)

- Cheech and Chong ("Man, that's false advertising")

- Berner (remember him?)

- Mike Tyson (I'm not saying shit, do your thing Iron Mike)

- Jaleel White (Urkel from Family Matters)

- Santana (say it ain't so Carlos!)

- Ooh LaLa (Run the Jewels, a contemporary "rap" group)

- B-Real (Cypress Hill sang "hits from the bong" hell of a song, rough lifestyle)

- Method Man (As high as Wu-Tang get)

- Jam Master Jay (Run-DMC brought hip-hop to the mainstream, arguably the most influential rap group in world history. JMJ was murdered in 2002 and his youngest son has a weed brand named after his dad)

- Lil Wayne (Same thing as that other young guy, in fact he and Wiz seem to be cut from the same millennial mold)

- Ricky Williams (NFL)

- Montel Williams (talk show guy)

- DJ Khaled (His song "all I do is win" went triple platinum, he is worth about $75m)

- CJ Wallace (The Notorious B.I.G's son. His dad was inducted into the rock and roll hall of fame in 2020 and went platinum 27 times, he is widely considered one of the greatest rappers of all time. His son has a weed brand)

- 2 Chainz (he was cited for possession the first time at 15 since has had plenty of drug related charges and convictions but never had jail time, in fact he was in a drug diversion program after being arrested for possession of lots of different drugs and multiple illegal firearms. The idea was to help him get better not punish him)

- Tiki Barber (NFL)

- Kevin Durant (NBA salary in 2023 will be $42.97m, his net worth is around $200m)

- Ghostface Killa (just too much of a fan to talk trash)

- Magic Johnson (We all know him, focused on CBD rather than THC)

*Drake and Whoopey Goldberg's brands have gone out of business

Now for a list of the white people making lots of money in the weed industry!

- Martha Stewart (seriously)

- Rob Gronkowski (duh)

- Seth Rogan (you're kidding)

- Willie Nelson ("When I die roll me up and smoke me")

- Jim Belushi (famous for being the brother of a famous actor, he impersonates his brother to sell the weed brand)

- Melissa Ethridge (singer)

The other white people invested in the weed industry are only famous if you read *The Wall Street Journal* every day. I you do read that kind of thing, you would be impressed with all the "celebrity investors." The Koch Brothers, for example, have annual combined revenues around $100 Billion. They began with lots of money from their dad, Fred. Fred was, according to many, a first class jerk, making his money from oil and building refineries. In 1934/35, Fred was in Germany pitching a refinery to the Third-Reich, in fact, he needed to get permission from Hitler himself. I doubt he had stage fright when kicking it with the Fuhrer because he had spent a bunch of years building refineries for Joseph Stalin! So the Koch empire was built, in part, thanks to Hitler and Stalin; now for the rest....

Much has been written and presented in documentaries about how the Koch brothers have increased their fortune by being ruthless. Here are some highlights: They stole oil from Native American reservations. Between '97 and '18 they spent over $145m attacking climate change science and solutions, voter suppression, responsible for over 300 oil spills, that kind of stuff.[16]

Anyway, the last remaining Koch, Charles, now loves THC, or at least the money that THC can bring him. On 4/6/21, Politico wrote an interesting article entitled: <u>"Koch-Backed Group Joins Marijuana Push After Zoom with Snoop Dogg."</u> As it turns out, Charles backs the idea of legalizing all drugs and would love to start with weed. Here is a quote from the article, emphasis mine: "Americans for Prosperity is excited to work alongside our partners to **bring cannabis businesses into the light, replacing black and gray markets with a free and fair legal framework,**" Brent W. Gardner, chief government affairs officer for Americans for Prosperity, said in a statement. **"Cannabis commerce will become a way for Americans to lift themselves up, rather than a barrier holding them back."**[17] This quote illustrates the emphasis on commerce over anything that resembles justice or ideals. Charles has lots of money but it isn't enough, the answer to him and his cohorts is "more," regardless of whom it hurts.

It is estimated that the commercial cannabis market in the US in 2023 will exceed $37 billion; $72 billion by 2030. I think that number is a little high but New Frontier doesn't:[18] (https://new-frontierdata.com/cannabis-insights/new-state-markets-could-boost-u-s-legal-cannabis-sales-to-72b-by-2030/)

In 2021 this country spent $27.9 billion on books. We spent about the same on cannabis that year. While book sales are pretty steady, weed sales are growing like crazy.[19] One has to wonder about the future of any nation that spends more money on getting high than reading. I propose that if the wealthy elite and celebrities spent their time and money advocating for a more educated and informed nation, it would happen. It would probably progress more slowly because education is not addictive, but the needle would be moved. The problem is that there isn't any money to be made advocating for knowledge, but there has always been a lot of money to be made selling intoxicating substances.

I hope that I am making my position more clear. I am not the anti-weed guy; I am the anti-corporate greed guy, the pro-recovery guy, and an advocate for common sense guy. Most of the issues could be fixed by getting rid of this industry. We want to change laws, cool. Let people grow and possess a personal amount. Get rid of the sharks who smell blood in the water. Corporate weed is evil!

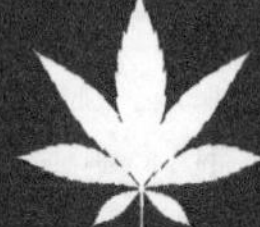

CHAPTER

03

THE POTENCY ISSUE AND TOLERANCE

Pushback met with Pushback

I talk about these things publicly. A new and common question has arisen in the last few years. Of all the stuff I say in a typical talk the one thing I can count on being asked is why people use concentrates. It is a moment in each presentation where I can tell who my fellow addicts are and who is "normal." If I play a video of people using concentrates and having an intense reaction, the vast majority of the room gasps and is like, "Why in the world would anyone do that!" The rest of the room, myself included, is like "Damn, I cant believe that I missed that stuff!" The addict's brain is not the same as others. We love extreme sensations and concentrates will deliver that reaction quickly. Addicts want to be gone from reality and concentrates also do that quickly, until they don't. So the first answer to the question, "Why do concentrates," is that the addict's brain thinks, if one pleasurable, escape reality substance is good, two is better. The second reason for concentrates has to do with tolerance.

Here is a helpful definition of tolerance: "Tolerance is a person's diminished response to a drug, which occurs when the drug is used repeatedly and the body adapts to the continued presence of the drug."[1]

The tolerance issue is closely tied to the "more is better" idea. Since a small minority of the consumers consume a majority of the THC, the market is dependent on the most frequent users.[2] Those users consume a lot of THC, an average of 1.35 grams a day![3] And as they use THC, they are building a tolerance to it. The idea is simple, so don't get side tracked by these unfamiliar words. Your body is full of cannabinoid receptors. Super high potency THC, as well as the increasingly frequent use of it, saturates those receptors and makes it harder and harder for those receptors to allow THC to bind to them. Add to this the reality that there is not a lethal overdose to THC; we have all heard "weed has never killed anyone." (See chapter in my previous book.) But you end up in a situation where the most addicted users ("most valuable users" in the eyes of the weed industry) can't feel the products they ingest unless they ingest much more and with much stronger potencies.

I need to be very clear about how this works, so let me illustrate with a narrative. (This narrative will have an accelerated time frame for brevity, tolerance does not happen this quickly.)

Eric is a grownup who smokes weed a couple of times a month. It isn't doing much harm. Eric voted 'yes' on Amendment 64 in Colorado, the law that allowed for commercial THC sales and was in line early on 1/1/14 when his local dispensary opened. In talking to the budtender (yes, that's what they're called) he realized how much he has been missing out on by smoking the same moderate weed for years. The budtender told him about the 6th most potent strain that was sold in 2014, something called "Death Star," tipping the scales at just under 24% THC. Eric was a bit unsure but got talked into it, bought some, went home and rolled one up. Three hits into the joint he was high as a kite and he loved it. The next day he woke up to the mostly unsmoked joint (he set it down when he got super high) and decided to take a hit or two even though it's a Sunday and he never smokes on Sundays. He remembered the awesome high from the day before and wants it again, after all he finally figured out what the song Maggot Brain by Funkadelic was all about. (Don't know that song? You're welcome.) This time it took Eric four hits to get the feeling he had the day before. After he burned through the Death Star he bought on day one, he went back to the same dispensary and told the same budtender how awesomely high he got. So the kid on the other side of the counter sold him the strongest strain of 2014, "Ghost Train Haze #1," coming in at a now moderate 27% THC, but a historical high water mark. Eric went home, rolled up the new bud and got as high as he did the first time, but this time it took four hits and he was smoking 3% stronger weed.

Let's skip forward a few years now and include some current products. Eric has been using THC daily for a long time now. He has a punch card that gives him rewards at several dispensaries. He also clips coupons (available in the local paper and in various kinds of publications widely available in grocery stores and and other businesses throughout town) and gets THC very cheaply. In spite of the cost-cutting, buying high potency "weed" is still a big part of his monthly spend (just what Arcview wants). He gets text messages from dispensaries, pop-up ads on his computer, direct mail and even invitations to events because he is such a good customer. Eric has tried to quit several times but never makes it more than a couple of days. He's always welcomed back to the dispensary with open arms. It is now 2022 and Eric has so saturated his endocannabinoid system that he is unable to feel anything at all unless he uses a concentrate. He vapes a 99.9% pure distillate multiple times a day, but never feels high; he just feels "normal" for a bit after using. He also uses edibles. He started back in 2014 with the occasional brownie, with 15% THC flower baked into it. Back then that was enough to get the feeling that he wanted to feel. Now he is eating a cake pop each day with 1000mg's of concentrate in each one (according to the packaging, that's 100 legal servings) to feel what he wants. Eric is exactly the consumer that the THC industry needs to grow and remain profitable. They make sure he is cradled and coerced, because he is always on the forefront of their minds and financial models. They will target him for the rest of his life with their products.

While the above narrative is fictional it is derived from hundreds of stories that I have heard, first-hand. They all follow a predictable trajectory, starting off slow and innocent, ending up in addiction and with a lower standard of living. Understanding the true nature of tolerance to THC will help us understand why commercial markets must move consumers towards concentrate use. The most profitable users will need those extremely potent products to feel any effect. This wouldn't be a bad thing if concentrates were healthy or even benign, but they are neither. These products are also very unregulated! Combine an unregulated market with a profitable and addictive substance and we have a recipe for trouble.

Now, let me tell you a story about a real person, her name is Dawn Reinfeld. Dawn is not someone you want to pick a fight with, I have said that the day I find myself facing her from the other side of an issue, I will run away and hide. She is tenacious, smart, well connected, and angry, with good cause.. A couple of years ago, addiction to THC hit close to home for Dawn so she started to look into it more. As a political insider who has fought for years as a Democrat activist, she had lots of friends she could call within the party to figure out how Colorado ended up where we did, pushing concentrates to kids. Dawn voted for medical marijuana but "felt lied to" when A64's push for recreational came around. She broke from her party and voted 'no' on 64. (I have great admiration for political people who think!) Dawn's research into the recreational weed industry led her to a mutual friend, we live in the same county, who introduced us. Within five minutes of our first telephone conversation, I knew I had found a kindred spirit. Dawn was talking about getting legislation together that would limit the industry's sales of concentrates and make it harder for healthy kids to get medical cards. I was excited but also felt the need to warn her that any attempt to limit the profits of the multi-billion dollar THC industry would be a street fight and that she would take some hard hits. Dawn didn't care, and still doesn't. While nobody likes having mean things written about them and being told they are trying to take medicine from sick and dying children, Dawn held to her well-researched truth and fought like hell. The result was HB (House Bill) 21-1317 "Regulating Marijuana Concentrates."[4] The bill was originally drafted to include a potency cap on PRODUCTS, a cap on THC flower without a cap on products is worth nothing. When consulted about where the cap should land, I went with the science: there is no safely established amount of THC. Research indicates that you lose medicinal value above 10% THC, and there is still very little research on "high potency" weed, over 16% THC.[5] Since we have plenty of solid evidence about the detrimental psychological and physical health issues associated with 16% and under, my suggestion was to cap products at 16%, if and until they could be proven safe.[6] When it became obvious that this idea was DOA, thanks to the dozens of lobbyists working for the THC industry, I suggested that we double that number to 32%. That percentage was not grounded in the science, but I thought doubling the highest amount we knew anything about would give the house bill a fighting chance at approval. Again, the industry didn't see it this way, they were thinking about Eric and how much harder it would be to keep making new "Erics" without their concentrates. Sitting in a room with a bunch of the industry people involved, I asked what kind of potency cap would be acceptable. I was met with blank stares, and then they told me, "None, we will not accept any cap." Afterall, they said, there is no proof that a 99.9% THC product is bad. I pointed to the research showing how bad things started to get around 12% and how they got worse between that and 16%. The lobbyists took the position that since there was not yet research on stuff that strong, there was no evidence that it was bad. Call me crazy but shouldn't the manufacturer have to prove that what they are selling is safe rather than the consumer prove that it is safe to consume? It's like saying no research has been done on how good or bad it is for a person to eat what's in the used kitty litter box every day, so by default it must be good for you! Let's carry this ridiculous illustration a bit further to prove a point. No one (that I know of) is feasting on cat poop every day, but if the state sanctioned the sale of cat poop and allowed it to be neatly packaged and sold in stores, wouldn't there be an implication that it was safe to eat? And why not make it available to children too? Afterall, there's no research saying it's not healthy!

There exists a social contract in this country under which the consumer assumes that things sold to them commercially are safe; there is also a legal obligation. In 1906, the Food and Drug Administration (FDA) was formed following the passage of the Federal Foods and Drugs Act. Prior to that, it was called "The Department of Chemistry." In 1938, the law was essentially replaced by a more comprehensive Food Drug and Cosmetic Act.[7] There have been a number of amendments/additions to this law, but it is still the governing principle. The importance of the FDA is pretty hard to overstate. Before its inception, people sold whatever they felt like selling and made whatever claims they wanted to make.[8] Samuel Hopkins Adams, in 1905, wrote an eleven-part article about all of the nonsense that was being sold as medicine and how much food with dangerous ingredients were sold. The public was outraged and demanded a change. People wanted assurance that medicines and foods were safe. Within a year, the

FDA was established. Here is an excerpt from the first of Mr. Adams' articles, emphasis mine:

"Gullible America will spend this year some seventy-five millions of dollars in the purchase of patent medicines. In consideration of this sum it will swallow huge quantities of alcohol, an appalling amount of opiates and narcotics, a wide assortment of varied drugs ranging from powerful and dangerous heart depressants to insidious liver stimulants; and far in excess of all other ingredients, undiluted fraud. **For fraud, exploited by the skillfulness of advertising bunco men, is the basis of the trade...***"*

Over the years since then, the FDA has played a larger and larger role in our society; keeping those "advertising bunco men" in check. For those of you not familiar with turn of the century slang, "bunco" means a cheat or con-man. Thanks to the efforts of the FDA over the past 115 years, we can have confidence and assume that things we are sold for consumption are safe and that things we purchase from a store are regulated according to reliable scientific and safety guidelines. But now we find ourselves in a world where billions of dollars of consumable goods are being sold with no FDA oversight. These goods are cannabis-based. The bunco men (and occasionally women) are laughing all the way to the bank, just like they did in times past. If we continue to accept the manufacturers' and their lobbyists' requirements that the consumer prove safety of products rather than their makers, then we will be taking a major step backwards and sacrificing the progress made over the years.

The Facts

There is no evidence that concentrates are safe, and I mean none. In March of 2021, a group of researchers from Colorado University in Boulder and Colorado State University in Fort Collins published a paper in the 2021 Australasian Professional Society on Alcohol and other Drugs, called "Advancing the science on cannabis concentrates and behavioral health." The excerpt below, from the paper's abstract, is revealing. I added the emphasis.

"The Cannabis sativa L. plant contains hundreds of phytocannabinoids, but putatively of highest importance to public health risk is the psychoactive cannabinoid delta-9-tetrahydrocannabinol (THC), which is associated with risk for cannabis use disorder, affective disturbance, cognitive harm and psychomotor impairment. Recently, there has been an increase in the use and availability of concentrated cannabis products (or concentrates) that are made by extracting cannabinoids from the plant to form a product with THC concentrations as high as 90 – 95%. These products are increasingly popular nation-wide. **The literature on these widely available high potency concentrates is limited and there are many unknowns about their potential harms.**"[10]

These authors systematically reviewed 185 published studies in order to present sound information on concentrate use, and guess what they found? First, they talked a bunch about tolerance and how that has led to an increased market for concentrates. They they addressed addiction (Cannabis use disorder) as well as the negative health effects. Not only do they not demonstrate or hint at any good that comes from concentrate use, but their conclusion states:

> *At present, we do not have sufficient data to make accurate conclusions about the severity of risks of these products. Gaps in the literature on their acute and long-term effects on human health need to be addressed in order to generate information about the effects of concentrates, in particular whether, and which forms, of these products are most harmful.*

Note this line in the conclusion; "...of these products are the most harmful." The researchers do not reference which of these products helps the most, rather what is the most harmful. These products are not safe! That is why HB1317 (mentioned earlier) mandated that each sale of a concentrate come with a warning, a big, 4-page warning. Hearing the industry representatives oppose this warning, claiming it was unnecessary and unjust, was appalling. At one point, a major criticism of the warning actually became the anticipated environmental impact of all that paper! For the sheer hypocrisy of this claim, please see my chapter on the environmental damages caused by the weed industry. The guy running the Colorado Cannabis Manufactures Association, Kevin Gallagher, was quoted in a local paper as saying "At the end of the day, these educational resources are going to litter our parking lots. We've got to print them out and fold them. It's laborious and cost-intensive, and just bad for the environment."[11] Sure, Kevin, this is about the trees! Perhaps the litter isn't their greatest worry, but it's more about the warnings contained within the handout, stuff like:

> "Warning Use of Marijuana Concentrate May Lead To: Psychotic Symptoms and or Psychotic disorder (Delusions, hallucinations of difficulty distinguishing reality). Mental Health Symptoms/Problems. Cannabis Hyperemesis Syndrome (CHS) uncontrolled and repetitive vomiting. Cannabis use disorder/dependence including physical and psychological dependence."[12]

RISKS AND PRECAUTIONS

WARNING:
Use of Marijuana Concentrate may lead to: [1]

1. Psychotic symptoms and/or Psychotic disorder (delusions, hallucinations, or difficulty distinguishing reality)[2];

2. Mental Health Symptoms/Problems[3];

3. Cannabis Hyperemesis Syndrome (CHS) (uncontrolled and repetitive vomiting);

4. Cannabis use disorder / dependence, including physical and psychological dependence.

**Consuming concentrate via inhalation
will cause immediate effects.**

Marijuana concentrates ARE NOT recommended for inexperienced marijuana users. THC concentration (% THC), amount of concentrate consumed, and frequency of use can result in both short and long-term effects. There is moderate evidence that individuals who use marijuana with THC concentration greater than 10% are more likely than non-users to be diagnosed with a psychotic disorder, such as schizophrenia.

Marijuana concentrate is not approved by the FDA and claims of medical benefits are not supported by the FDA.

Marijuana concentrates ARE NOT recommended for anyone under age 25, except if recommended by a doctor. People 25 and under may be at greater risk of potential harm because the brain is not fully developed.

Regulated Marijuana Stores cannot provide medical advice. Any questions related to the health or safety of marijuana concentrates should be discussed with a patient's recommending physician or an adult consumer's primary care physician.

[1] These risks are based on CDPHE evidence statements where there is either moderate or substantial evidence. Where moderate means strong scientific findings that support the outcome, but these findings have some limitations and substantial means robust scientific findings that support the outcome with no credible opposing scientific evidence. https://marijuanahealthinfo.colorado.gov/glossary

[2] When associated with other risk factors, including psychiatric history.

[3] When associated with other risk factors, including psychiatric history.

2

The pamphlet also comes with a suggested serving size, which is "about half the size of a grain of rice," and a pictorial illustration of how large that actually is. The pamphlet also has the phone numbers and websites for Rocky Mountain Poison Control and the National Suicide Hotline. The weed industry knows

that telling people a serving is a tiny amount and to giving consumers a number to call if they feel suicidal or feel like they were
poisoned will not be helpful to their bottom line and reputation.
The pamphlet also includes this startling warning: "This product
was produced without regulatory oversight for health, safety or
efficacy."

I am going to be very direct here; concentrates have no place in
the human brain or body, none. There is ample proof that they
are unsafe and there exists no evidence that they are in any way
safe. Yet they have a huge place in the commercial market. Concentrate weed products are extremely profitable and essential to
the industry in order to satisfy the increasing tolerance demands
of their biggest consumers.

What we are seeing is a classic science vs economics scenario.
What we have seen demonstrated again and again (opiates, tobacco, etc) is that economics will win in the short term and eventually
science and truth will rule the day, sadly, after much irreversible
damage has been done. The fundamental question is, "How long
will it take America this time to put facts and truth over bunco
artists, disguised as business people, and greed?"

The chapter would have ended here if I didn't sit down with
Dawn for a couple of hours to talk about HB 1317. She had some
really important stuff to share and this feels like the right place.

Sitting in her backyard, on a perfect Colorado fall day, I asked
her a few questions. First, why would anyone in their right mind
decide to pick this fight. Her answer was insightful, "The State
Legislature was disconnected, they didn't know what was happening in the real world or what was being sold in the shops
they were supposed to be regulating." Dawn saw an issue and had
faith in the political process to resolve it. She went on to tell me
how almost every single person in her peer group has had high
potency THC issues in their personal/family lives. She figured it
would be easy to get a group of angered voters together around
these issues, she was right! Her PAC, "Blue Rising," set a goal of
getting legislation passed that would have a science-based poten-

cy cap, and she knew that would have to be a compromise. Again, Dawn knows how the process works. Blue Rising also wanted to tighten up the "medical" designation process. Dawn told me that one of the most frustrating things about this whole situation was how THC had no explicit criteria regarding its medical properties. THC has no dosage amounts, no duration of effectiveness, no limits, and it is exceptionally easy for 18 year olds to get their medical access cards. Dawn figured that if it was going to be medicine or at least treated like we treat alcohol, then it should be regulated.

To kick things off, Dawn and a few friends, the Colorado Attorney General (AG), a middle school dean, the Boulder District Attorney (DA), a therapist, and a coalition of parents, put on an educational session at the State capital, publicizing it to everyone there for weeks. When the day finally came, Dawn estimated that 3-4 lawmakers actually attended. Several sent Aids and a few stopped by, grabbed the free food and left. One of the lawmakers who did show was Democratic representative to the House, Yadira Caravero. Dr Caravero is a pediatrician and she paid very close attention. Despite the bagel spread, placed literally outside of the door of the session and sponsored by the cannabis industry, Dr. Caravero sat through the presentation, asked questions, afterwards did her research, and then offered to sponsor the bill. It is telling that the only physician in the Legislature stepped forward and asked Dawn to sponsor what would be HB 1317. Additional key sponsors would end up being none less than the Speaker of the House, Alec Garnet, Chris Hansen, the chair of the Appropriations Committee, and Paul Lundeen, the Republican Whip. The bill was also sponsored by a bi-partisan partnership between Republican Tim Geitner and Democrat Kevin Priola, and 28 co-sponsors. HB 1317 passed with overwhelming support, and very little opposition. However, the pushback and strong resistance came from the industry, which fought and lobbied and fought some more. In the end, they delayed the potency cap. Despite the Colorado Association of School Executives saying "you will not find one district in the state that will not support 1317," our old friend Mason Tvert, Colorado's biggest carpetbagger, was quoted as saying the Bill is "a heavy-handed attempt to move the clock back to an era of prohibition." It's pretty incredible to believe an attempt to determine and implement true evidence based regulations is called prohibition. Reactions like this, irrational and self-serving, is what Mason and others have used to build their careers and empires.

Dawn told me story after story of crazy stuff that happened throughout her efforts to hold the weed industry accountable; none surprising but all frustrating. We talked for a long time enjoying the weather and conversation. As we were wrapping up I asked one last question; if she thought this would become more of a Democrat issue in the future, given that it was about health and wellness as well as challenging big corporate influence. She thought for a bit and gave a very thoughtful answer. "We can't be the party of drugs," she said, explaining that it all started with good intentions. She believes her party intended to reform a broken justice system and address racism in the legal process. Most politicians, she said, wanted to do the right thing; "I didn't see corruption, I saw uninformed people." She thought that by showing lawmakers the products being sold and consumed many will be shocked into action. "The courage of the parents and kids who shared their stories was what did it, we just need to help them feel okay about speaking up and stick with them when they do." Dawn stopped talking for a minute while watching the dogs chase falling leaves in the yard and feeling the breeze that was just rolling in. Then, with tears in her eyes, Dawn turned to me and spoke, for her this is all so very real. She told me that the stories she heard from parents and kids moved her deeply. There were stories of addiction and psychosis, of the young lady who was incapacitated after using concentrates and raped, the alternative school kids who all spoke of the devastation concentrates have left in their lives and among their peers, and all of the parents who had to watch helplessly as their kids' lives spiraled out of control, realizing what they were using was much more than "just weed." "As long as people keep speaking up and we keep supporting them when they do, this will be way more than a Democrat issue, it will be a human issue." Well said Dawn!

Bottom line is this: for-profit sales lead to a focus on the frequent user, the frequent user builds tolerance, and tolerance demands stronger products; a market in which concentrates rule. Is this ultimately about making money or about ideals, like personal freedom and responsibility for one's choices? Ask the person arguing for legalized "commercialization" if they would support a potency cap. True believers in the benefits of the plant and those who care about social justice won't care, but the big business exploiters will balk at the idea. They need addiction to finance their lifestyles, lawyers, and marketeers; guys like Mason Tvert don't come cheap.

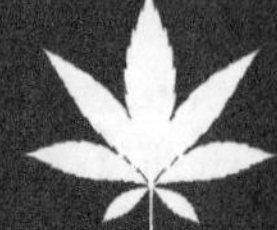

CHAPTER

04

BLACK MARKET

We made it stronger on all fronts. The logic of hurting cartels by legalizing this drug only ends with legalizing everything, like everything.

I remember being at a debate or town hall or something back when we were talking about A64 in Colorado. At one point a fellow stood up and said something to the effect of, "I'm not into the idea of weed, but if we can do anything at all that hurts the cartels, even a tiny little bit, I will vote for it, so I'm voting 'yes'." He then went on to talk about how evil the cartels are and some awful graphic stories about stuff they have pulled in the past. He was passionate and fired people up about the awful actions of the cartels. I tried to make the point that hating cartels didn't mean we should support commercialized weed. Global warming sucks too, but that has nothing to do with Amendment 64. Many of us had long insisted just the opposite, that allowing for recreational THC sales would only strengthen cartels. Not only would there be more users, they wouldn't be paying taxes and would benefit from the widening use without higher overhead costs. Think about it, the cartels no longer had to smuggle tons (literal tons) of product across the border, they just had to get a few people here to set up shop. Not only did they do that right away, they were able to switch their distribution channels from the south and from weed to much more profitable things, like meth and opiates. We need look no further than the overdose rates these past few years as well as what is being intercepted at the border to understand that legalization helped the cartels increase their business. They are growing weed all over the US, but the black market has exploded, bringing up more and stronger drugs than ever before. The anti-cartel talking point made simple sense, as long as people didn't actually understand how they work. For anyone willing to consider the realities, that argument fell flat. We now have more than enough evidence to prove this, will we listen?

I have long advocated that the best way to actually hurt cartel bottom lines is to reduce use, and I mean the use of all drugs that they sell, not just weed. What most people fail to realize is that someone with a substance use disorder (the best customers and biggest consumers) very rarely abuse one substance. The goal of the addict is intoxication/escape/comfort, and it doesn't matter whether it's THC or meth or fentanyl. The people who sell intoxicating drugs want people to use any and all of them because that increases the chance that they will use the particular drug that they provide. We must also remember that there is no "weed cartel." Drug cartels are just that, drugs, lots of drugs and not just one specific kind of drug. If we diminish one of their drug sales channels they will just expand to another. I'm pretty sure that the cartels are thinking, "This is fantastic! America has legal weed so it's time to start growing it up there and shift operations down here to make meth and Fentanyl!"

The "Rocky Mountain High Intensity Drug Trafficking Area" is the agency that fights black market drugs, all drugs, and they keep pretty good records. In their Fall 2020 report we can see a pretty clear trend.[1] In 2014, 5215 cannabis plants were seized. Every year since then, the numbers have only risen: in 2015, 14,979; in 2016, 47,108; in 2017, 48,325; in 2018, 60,026; in 2019, 68,600; and in 2020, 86,502. Those numbers DO NOT indicate a struggling black market, they indicate a thriving and growing black market, AFTER legalization.

Now let's look at the same numbers for overdose deaths in Colorado following legalization:[2]

In 2015, the year after A64 passed, 880 people died from drug overdose. In 2016, there were 912 deaths; in 2017, 1,012; in 2018, 974; in 2019, 1,072; and in 2020, the highest number of OD's were recorded, 1,477. Anybody else seeing a problem here? I wonder if we are doing any better nationally on OD's in light of the increased legalized access?[3]

In 2015, 52,623 lost their lives; in 2016, there were 63,938 deaths; in 2017, 70,699; in 2018, 67,850; in 2019, 71,130; and in 2020, 92,478 died, a 30% increase in just a year! Right before this went to publication we got some FBI data showing an increase in cannabis-related arrests from 2021-2022. In '21 there were

219,489 total arrests and in '22 that rose to 227,108. Not only has the black market increased, but arrests are still rising.[4]

I'm not saying that one has led to the other, well I kind of am; what I am saying is that this isn't working. We tried a war on drugs, which traded high use rates for high incarceration rates, so that didn't work. Most recently we tried this whole commercialization thing, and if we're honest about those facts, that clearly isn't working. How about a war on stupid! In this war we would hold accountable those people who oversimplify complex issues into inaccurate and harmful sound bites. We would seriously penalize people who put corporate greed and profit over public health. The first likely result of this proposed war is that many politicians and the nation's lobbyists would be under investigation. The upside is that you could sell tickets to go visit them to offset the costs. People could pay to observe them all in cages and on special days see them get fed. I for one would like to see them throwing poo at one another. I urge that we consider putting that prison/zoo somewhere in New Jersey because, well, New Jersey.

Back to the cartels and organized crime. In order to truly dent their margins we need to take away all of their drug sales, perhaps by making all drugs legal and as safe as possible. Let me be clear, that I am not advocating. Imagine the establishment and implementation of national standards we discussed for testing potency and purity of marijuana and multiply it by a lot. The need for additional governmental infrastructure to handle such an undertaking would be as big as anything we have undertaken since building highways. That would probably lose support from the Libertarians, they aren't too into expanding government. On the other hand, the Republicans will probably like it because it's more tax money from industry and the Democrats will like more government oversight.

The other option, and one I prefer, is to lower demand for drugs within the American population. Why is it that the United States population gets so much "higher" than other countries?[5] If we were just a nation that liked to have a good time people would stop at that rather than go on to addiction as a means of self-medicating mental illness. As someone who had limited access to mental health services when I was in my darkest times, I believe that we end up treating our pain and illness however we can. Nobody wants to hurt, be that physically or emotionally. If I had access to care and took advantage of it, I have to assume that my drug use would have been much less and maybe never graduated to addictive use. We can't simply tell people who are hurting, desperate, hopeless to "just say no" without giving them solutions to get better. With well-funded mental health stigma-reducing campaigns, as well as access to effective care, I believe that we could reduce the need for people to self-medicate with illicit and unproven substances; substances that often magnify the core issues while just masking symptoms. Only treating symptoms may make people into good, returning "customers," but the goal should be on wellness.

The hippie side of me will reveal itself later in the chapter on environmental issues, but here's a bit of a preview. Cartels in the US do not play by EPA standards. Oregon and CA have had a glut of cartel grows pop up on public lands.[6] There are plenty of issues with this, such as the significant impact on soil, water and wildlife. More about that later.

Just looking at the sheer numbers of busts in the years since legalization, is another illustration of how well this is not working to damage cartels.[7] Until we are prepared to actually do what it takes to regulate all drugs, to build the infrastructure for their sale to be as safe as possible, a momental task that we are clearly not up to, drug cartels will continue to flourish. While the individual effect will be nothing, the aggregate could be real. If enough of us stopped getting high, or even got less high, they would feel it.

The reality is that we don't produce cocaine in the US and we produce MUCH less meth than in years past. These products come from Central and South America and more and more of our illicit opioid supply also comes from south of the border.[8,9] Those who use these substances directly support the cartels and indirectly they reinforce their violent and oppressive actions. Since people who use THC are more likely to use these other substances as well, the higher the THC use in America the better their business will be down South.[10] Recently an article has been making the rounds telling us that for the first time in US history more people are using THC than smoking cigarettes.[11] Not only is this exciting news for the Big Weed producers in this country, it is for the cartels as well. More THC use leads to more use of their other substances. Every one of the substances they sell has blood on it. Let's stop kidding ourselves, higher drug use will be good only for people who sell the drugs.

On 12/16/22 a guy named Mike Bebernes wrote a story called "Why Hasn't Legal Weed Killed the Marijuana Black Market?" The article's author cites a report out of LA showing that illegal grows outnumber legal by as much as 10/1 in California. There are plenty of noteworthy points made in the article but let me provide one well researched quote from it "The proliferation of illegal pot farms has also brought with it a surge in violent crime, human trafficking, and severe environmental damage in the areas where unlicensed growing is concentrated."[12] Another recent article highlighted how the Sinaloa Cartel is getting into the legal weed business. The article quotes one of the cartel's producers saying "We are buying seeds from all over the world to create our own strain, to produce top notch Sinaloa weed and to develop a strong brand even better than the gringos." He goes on to say that "the Juniors," El Chapo's sons, are investing in lobbying with Mexico's top politicians to legalize weed.[13]

So lets make sure that we have this straight; the cartels are giving money to and lobbying for legal weed Nice work DPA and NORML, you guys really messed up on this one. In a shortsited and misguided attempt to grab some more money, these American Special interests have aligned politically with the Sinaloa Cartel and likely others. Had people taken the time to "play the movie out," as we say in AA, they would have seen this inevitable conclusion.

At this point we can either continue playing the "I can't see you game" and ignore all of this or we can actually take a hard look at why we get so high in America and what we could do to actually reduce the demand for drugs that cartels will always be there to meet.

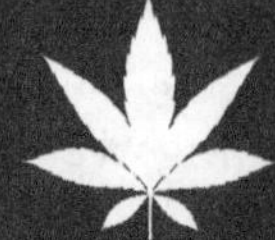

CHAPTER

05

FEDS

I'm guessing that the title originally suggested for this chapter won't make the final cut. It was kind of profane; just imagine some profanity and a reference to impotence. The Federal Government is asleep at the wheel on these matters. In fact, they are not just asleep at the wheel, they are letting kids drive while they sleep. The feds regulate medicine and food as well as other intoxicants, like alcohol and cigarettes. Since they have decided that hands-off is the best approach with THC, regulating the multi-billion dollar weed market is left to the states who have no infrastructure for doing so. Since states do not have the experience or the resources necessary to effectively regulate this market, they do a poor job at it. They all talk a big game, like a kid who wants to drive but can't, insisting they can get the job done but none (I repeat, none) have done so. If the American people want legal THC sales then the feds need to drive that train. The problem is that I doubt all the branches of government can find consensus on weed regulations. (Sometimes I wonder if they can agree on what day of the week it is!) Ted Cruz or AOC or somebody would start arguing that we use the wrong calendar or something like that. Then they'd get their pundit crew to agree just to fight. If we asked the tip-top fellas, at least as I write, Biden wouldn't remember what day it actually was and Trump would insist that it was Donaldday. Sadly and inexcusably, most of the people in DC wouldn't know a concentrate from a topical CBD cream. I blame the voters as much as I blame them because we are the ones who keep them in office, rather than demanding some accountability.

Since I believe that there are actually smart and compassionate people in DC, a few at least, I would like to spell out exactly how we could fix this mess at the Federal level. I will keep it simple and brief.

Most importantly and before anything else, we need to agree on a potency cap; identifying how strong is too strong must be considered. I have some experience helping states and other countries tackle this issue, and it's tough. It always comes down to this: the industry says any limit is too much while the doctors and scientific community say any amount is too much. We are going to have to find a compromise in order to set limits.

Whenever a politician kicks people out of the office and closes the door you know it's going to get good. Getting to see them when nobody is watching or recording is way fun. It's also a position that is earned when they know that you know how to shut up about things. For that reason I'm going to be vague. A state lawmaker once closed the doors to his office. After expressing his frustration with the THC lobby, he asked me where the science would likely land on the potency question. I laughed a bit and asked him if it really mattered; if there would be the political willpower to adhere to sound science. He told me he was optimistic but would need to know the numbers before he could say more. I told him that the best he could hope for was about 8% THC as a safe-ish and therapeutic amount and that it would have to contain a good deal of CBD. He leaned back in his chair and said "Well @@##, that's absolutely impossible." I agreed, the industry would never allow a limit so low. They know that 8% would result in a fraction of the addictive use and consequently, fewer profits. I then went on to tell him that any cap at all would be better than the current situation. The math is really simple, the lower the THC amount allowed, the less addiction to and mental illness from THC we will see. Incidentally, the lower the cap the fewer people we will need to treat at my program for cannabis use disorder, I am absolutely advocating for something that would negatively affect my bottom line, because there are more important things than the bottom line. You hear that THC guys, THERE ARE MORE IMPORTANT THINGS THAN THE BOTTOM LINE!

I advocate for a limit that is as close to zero as possible. The industry will argue for a limit that is as close to 100% as possible. We must find a point of agreement. My hope is that we spend more time thinking about what the doctors are saying rather than what the industry is feeding us. That requires keeping the money grabbers out of the room in which we decide how they will be regulated. The "wild-west" style standards that play out across the nation are a joke. Potency is not considered because the industry won't allow it. As of this writing, there exists a law or two limiting the potency of grown cannabis. While people want to call that a "potency cap" it is nothing of the sort because those plants are turned into products that are not governed by a cap. If THC in a plant is capped at 30%, it can still be turned into a concentrate with unlimited potency. That in turn can be infused into an edible, and none of those products have established caps. While a lower potency organic substance (flower) will require more refining and therefore more biomass it is still extremely cheap and easy to refine into the desired potency. We must also remember that no one is testing the plants being grown in the couple of places that have potency caps in a meaningful way. Before anything else is considered, a cap on potency must be established. If future sound science shows that it should be higher, make it so, if lower, make it so.

Next thing that needs to be tackled are the pesticides and fertilizers used in the growing of cannabis. It should be simple; since these products are being ingested, apply the same standards FDA requires for other things we take into our bodies. Currently, states do have limits on pesticides and heavy metals but they have a hard time enforcing their limits. This goes back to the earlier point that states don't have the resources to do the federal government's job. By shifting this responsibility to where it belongs much will be solved, or at least solved on paper. Regulation without enforcement is worthless, but we will get to that. There are pesticides and growth accelerators being used on cannabis that are not approved for topical exposure on animals, but humans are ingesting them orally and often combusting and inhaling them.[1]

Lastly, we need to give some very serious thought to the growing process and the byproducts created by such a large scale industry. What will they do with waste water? Will they have energy restrictions? (More details later about the high energy demands required to grow weed.)

73

So far, we have potency, toxins and environmental issues to consider. Once national regulations are determined, much thought must be given to how those regulations will be enforced. Enforcement is a logistical Mt. Everest, but I promised to keep this simple and brief so here goes!

The first enforcement challenge is determining what constitutes a representative sample to be tested. This hasn't been done before but I suggest around 5%. Who knows what 5% would be nationally but I did some napkin math based on 2020 Colorado numbers. In that year Colorado grew/sold about 1.46 million pounds of cannabis and our population was about 5.77 million.[2,3] That same year the US population was around 331 million. If the nation consumed at the same rate as Colorado that would amount to approximately 85 million pounds of weed. Five percent of that would be about 4,250,000 pounds set apart for testing. Although the problem is complex, let's just use these numbers to keep it simple.

The 4.25 million pounds of weed would need to be tested in federally certified labs operating under universal standards; 10% THC in Montana needs to be the same thing as 10% THC in New York. The next issue is how quickly those labs can make their determinations. Products can't go to market before they are determined to be safe and meet standards. Since weed manufacturers won't want to wait months before they can sell their products, plenty of labs and people to work in them will be needed in order to make the testing process quick and accurate. Now, who pays for all of this? It seems reasonable that the manufacturers bear that responsibility. If the cost includes taxes paid on their products, the consumer would also share the burden. Since this will likely be a big investment and require large annual expenditures, we will need to establish the cost to build the necessary infrastructure. After those costs are determined, it makes sense to require money from those hoping to be licensed, well in advance of sales so that things are in place before selling begins. Consequently, licensing fees need to be paid several years before retail sales open. Unfortunately, only the really big players will be able to make that kind of investment and be assured of getting a solid return. Now we're back to the troublesome issue of incentivizing weed sales to problem users to maintain high profits. In addition, 5% will be shaved off their bottom line because that product will be lost to testing, and shave off the licensing fees to establish the infrastructure. Their profit margins will take a substantial hit. Since making money is the driving force behind this industry, I would expect some serious pushback!

Enforcement at the local level, on growing operations and retail is next on the list. If you look at the complexity of the laws on the books in various states right now, you will quickly end up scratching your head wondering how in the world all those regs will be enforced. After all, a law is only as good as enforcement of that law. Since laws at the local and state level require various levels of enforcement, it is highly unlikely that anything will be done making sure the seed to sale tracking is working, let alone addressing the secondary issues of waste water, garbage (yes, that's a thing), smell pollution, chemicals used, and qualifications of the staff and owners. If we agree that the enforcement should be coming from the feds, all of these issues should be handled by a federal agency with local departments all over the country. I propose making the Bureau of Alcohol Tobacco and Firearms (AFT) the ATF&M. The Bureau of Alcohol Tobacco and Firearms is the most likely agency under which to roll marijuana enforcement. They have the infrastructure that could be expanded to include marijuana.

The question that all of this begs is one of taxes. How much will this product be taxed to make sure that costs are covered and hopefully, still have a bit left over? The common thinking in academic circles is probably around 30%. If you go much higher there's the probability that the black market will rule the day. If taxes are much lower, it's not cost-effective. By way of example, Colorado's nicotine tax is on its way up to 62% in the coming years.[4] That works because nicotine is so addictive and there is almost no black market; we shut that business down quickly. People are always going to buy smokes and drive them across the state line where they are cheaper, but organized crime doesn't work in that market much. THC may be another matter, but we won't really know until we try because taxing vice substances has always been tricky, from tobacco to booze to gambling. As a rule, more money is typically lost then made when all of the societal costs are considered. We also know that higher tax rates, and thereby prices, lead to lower youth use; that math is simple.[5] The trick with weed is that it's easy to grow and it's already well established in the criminal distribution system. If the tax rate is too high, it will lead to a huge portion of the market being controlled by organized crime and small-time growers/dealers. I suggest starting at a 30% tax rate and reassessing at preset intervals. By the way, if weed production and consumption were really about personal freedom and use, we could allow people to grow their own and not sell any. But in that scenario, there is no big money to be made, so it's probably never going to happen.

Amendment 64 (Colorado's recreational weed law) has preloaded fines that are so low they are laughable. Obviously, those fines were established by those who intended to sell, and not all of it selling above board.[6] To assure that fines are taken seriously and not just another acceptable cost of doing business, I believe that violations should be accompanied by rapidly ascending penalties. For instance, the first fine would be as much a warning as anything else. The second one would hurt, and the third would make them seriously consider changing their ways because their bottomline suffers. Since vertical integration and mergers and acquisitions are the norm in the business world, I recommend linking the fines directly to the profits of the business; big players pay more. Rather than set fines, charge a percentage of their gross profits for the month or quarter. This kind of financial penalty will motivate manufacturers and retailers to pay attention to the laws governing them.

Here is another crazy idea, but it just might work….. Since we can theoretically track cannabis plants using RFID tags from seed to sale, let's start doing it! If we commit to doing this (and the industry says they are committed), we can determine the origins of any illicit weed. That kind of Illicit weed is most often found in the hands, pockets, and stash boxes of minors. If we test every single product that is confiscated from minors, then we can penalize the growers/retailers because their product founds its way to kids. The industry will talk with passion about not wanting children and youth to get their products, but those are lies; the same kind tobacco companies used. If the weed industry is truly sincere about protecting kids from using their products, have them pay into a fund for youth prevention and treatment when their products are found on kids. The industry won't like this suggestion either. They want all of the profits and none of the responsibility. They are making money hand over fist in this "green rush." It's high time (no pun intended) they lose a little of that profit to offset the damage their products do.

The main point here is that 'regulating' isn't easy and I am sick of the people with the least interest in actual regulation (the industry) telling us that it's working great. Let's get them out of the room where this stuff is being decided and make them play by rules similar to everything else in this country that is sold commercially. No more special treatment for Big Marijuana!

Now that that is all out of the way, let's talk about rich politicians getting richer. Take outspoken pot proponent Nancy Pelosi, someone who regularly votes on THC related laws. In addition to owning an impressive portfolio of pot stocks, her son is the chairman of the board of "Freedom Leaf," now called by the rather ambiguous name, "GL Brands." It is a massive multi-national company involved in everything from hemp to concentrate extractions. Is that ethical? Can we make a world where the people making the laws don't get to cash in on those laws?

I could spend a full chapter talking about nepotism and the double standards among many inside the weed industry. Consider, for instance, Toi Hutchinson. She was the top cannabis enforcement official in Illinois for less than two years before taking a job heading up a national pro-weed lobby group that wrote the laws in that state and in many others. She is currently president and CEO of The Marijuana Policy Project or MPP. Then there's Andrew Freedman, Colorado's first "marijuana czar." He left that post to become a senior vice president at Forbes and Tate Partners, a DC-based lobbying firm that reported $14.5m in revenue in 2019 and works for groups like Altria (the cigarette and THC people) and a ton of big pharma companies.[7] Andrew is also the Executive Director of The Coalition for Cannabis Policy, Education and Regulation, another big pro-weed lobby group. How about Brian Pierce and Vincent Brown? They were lobbyists for the THC industry in Michigan who just got arrested, charged and convicted of federal crimes for bribing the then chair of the Michigan Marijuana Licensing Board. Or Ricardo Baca, who was our nation's first mainstream cannabis journalist when he took that job with the Denver post. Bacca now runs a cannabis marketing and advertising firm called "Grasslands." It makes its money helping THC manufacturers make more money. Does it make you wonder how objective his journalism was while at the post?

This list could go on and grow into its own chapter, but I'll leave it with these few examples and urge that we set some serious limits on those who regulate this substance and their ability to turn around and sell it. Also, we should push for a little more honesty in the journalism sector covering Big Pot.

Now, let's talk about research. The feds control the dollars that allow much of the meaningful research conducted in this country. They need to apply a significant amount of those dollars and resources into accurate and honest research of THC and CBD; into the efficacy and harms of this plant and its components. It is certainly possible to determine what is really safe and what is dangerous. After all, we can manufacture medicines, when warranted, and slap federal warning labels on things, when warranted. With some real investment into research, this conversation could finally move out of the dark ages where passion rules the day and into the 21st century where reason and genuine concerns for wellness are the chosen values.

In summary, I have sat in enough back rooms and spoken to more than enough politicians to be pretty sure that they are, for the most part, pretty damn basic. It seems that understanding these issues and committing to do what is right in the face of the powerful interests of the weed industry are not high priorities unless it adds to votes or personal enrichment. It is truly up to us to hold them accountable for their decisions, but we have failed when it comes to weed. I am not a one issue voter, but I make a point to know where those I am voting for stand on this issue. It factors immensely into where I donate and how I vote. Enough is enough, it's time for those in positions of authority, especially at the Federal level, to get off your self-serving, well-fed, privileged backsides and take some responsibility on this issue. Your inaction is making our lives harder. With this I close the chapter on federal politics, as well as any hope of ever having friends in government!

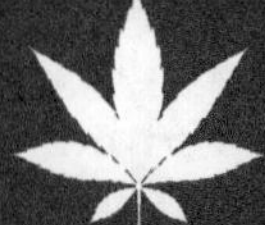

CHAPTER

06

WORKPLACE SAFETY AND DRIVING

It's still impossible to test

I like to stay busy. When not working with addicts in treatment or early recovery, writing, talking to athletes, lecturing, hanging with my family or fishing, I spend a good deal of time working with organized labor. For years I have been involved with Labor Assistance Professionals (LAP). LAP is a nonprofit, "dedicated to obtaining comprehensive alcohol and drug treatment and mental health services for our members at a reasonable and fair price." These fantastic people, connected to the labor movement and focused on the mental health and well-being of their members, do life changing work.[1] For years I have worked with specific unions helping them build policy aimed at helping members in need and educating their leadership and members on addiction and mental health issues. Over the last few years much of what I do with them has been focused on the damage caused by weed. This is important because most of their labor takes place in a safety-sensitive environment where everyone is at an elevated risk if anyone is intoxicated. Since so many of their locals are now located within weed "legal" states, measuring impairment has become crucial. THC does lots of things to the brain and body, some we know well, some we just suspect. A couple of things that we know well are that THC has an acute and immediate effect on a person's depth perception, on their singularity of focus, their ability to retain information, a slowing down of reaction time and it impairs motor coordination.[2] In many ways it is not unlike lots of other intoxicating substances that people can use after work but not during work. The trick with THC is that there is no test to determine intoxication. Tests can only show if THC is present in a person's system. This means that just because someone tests positive for THC does not mean that they are intoxicated, but they might be....

Here is the scenario I describe to classes I teach for unions, entitled "Welcome to Weed Country."

Chris and I are sheet metal workers and proud members of local 9 out of Denver. One Friday I ask Chris to join me for a cookout and fire in the backyard. Chris accepts and comes over on Saturday afternoon. While grilling I ask Chris if he wants to burn a joint with me. "Ha," says Chris "I haven't smoked since the 80's. Why not, it's legal now!" Knowing he will have no tolerance, I dig out some ditch (old-school low potency homegrown weed) weed, roll one up and we smoke before dinner. Later that night Chris catches an Uber home because he isn't stupid enough to drive high. He wakes up, laughs about the night before and goes on with his weekend. I wake up and follow my normal routine of using THC several times throughout the day and staying consistently high. Come Monday morning, I hit my vape pen several times on the way into work and, just because it's Monday, I eat a few gummies before heading in; it helps to make the day suck less. When Chris and I see one another at the morning meeting, I am stoned out of my mind and he is stone cold sober. There is no scenario in which Chris would still be intoxicated from Saturday, and there is no scenario under which I am sober and safe to work in a construction zone. Shortly into our work day there is an accident. To make a point, let's say I am the cause of the accident while working alongside sober Chris. The accident triggers a mandatory drug test and we both come up hot for THC. According to the single urinalysis (UA) test that we are both given, there is no difference between my urine and his; we are both "high."

Let's start with the easy truth, it is nonsense that Chris gets punished for being high on the job when he is not. In the same way that it would be nonsense for me to have no accountability for being high on the job when I am. The issue is that we do not, and there is little hope that we ever will, have a test to distinguish between Chris and myself. Since we cannot tolerate intoxication in the workplace the only solution is that we both must be able to demonstrate a "negative" test for THC on every single work day. The same principle exists for driving. Expecting those operating cars or machines to be sober is a right, using THC is a privilege; rights trump privileges. It's understandable that zero THC in one's system is far from a perfect solution but until someone invents a way to tell Chris from me, it is the only solution.

A couple of years ago, I was in a NFL locker room explaining the league's testing policy to players when one of them brought up the injustice of being punished for using a substance on their own time when it had nothing whatsoever to do with practice or games. I agreed with him in theory and pointed out that he was not required to play professional football. If using THC was a priority that was fine, he could use as much as he wanted just not be employed with the NFL. The same truth carries over for workers in safety sensitive positions and drivers. They get to choose based on their priorities, but your desire to use THC does not outweigh our collective right to safety. Without the equivalent of a .08 for THC, as exists for alcohol, the only way to determine sobriety is the total absence of THC.

Echoing the same case I made in my 2017 book, the economic incentives to create a test are so profound that the absence of such a test illustrates the immense difficulty of creating this test. The person who brings a reliable THC test to market that can determine intoxication will be racing helicopters with Jeff Bazos, Warren Buffet and Elon Musk. Here are some of the challenges facing anyone attempting to create such a test.

First, THC is fat soluble meaning that the half life is totally unpredictable unless you factor in body mass index, metabolism, age, sex and use history. Second, blood is not a reliable form of testing because THC works its way out of your bloodstream and into your glucose (brain juice) in less than an hour. Unless we test brain fluid (hard to do on the living), that idea is out. Third, intoxication limits are not set in stone. For instance, The arbitrary measurement of 5ng/ml of THC in blood that Colorado set as the legal driving limit is worthless because it has been demonstrated in court multiple times that under that limit does not mean sober and over the limit does not mean intoxicated.[4]

For a while, Hound Labs "breathalyzer" that could measure use within about 3 hours, seemed like a new, interesting, and helpful idea.[5] Concerning was the shortness of the 2-3 hour window since impairment has been measured up to 24 hours after use.[6] The biggest drawback is financial; each testing unit is around $5k per and processing is $20/test after that. The more significant issue however lies in the fact that many people are not smoking let alone using THC orally. This is described in detail in the next chapter, "What Can't They Do." Given how easy it is to get intoxicated from THC in ways that do not require inhaling combusted cannabis solutions that measure only that will never suffice.

We put the cart ahead of the horse on this one. Prior to legal sales, a quick and affordable way of measuring impairment must be determined.

There is a new issue that is starting to spring up around the country as more and more states allow THC use, and that is pre employment testing. While the vast majority of states still allow for this to take place there are some exceptions.[7]

- California

  Testing is only permitted for positions of sensitivity in state agencies if testing is job related. Testing is required for public transportation drivers.

- Montana

  Testing permitted for applicants to intrastate transport jobs, hazardous environments jobs, or positions with security, public safety, or fiduciary responsibility.

- Nevada

  Testing ONLY permitted for public safety jobs

- New Jersey

  Testing permitted, but employers cannot refuse to hire any person because they do (or do not) use cannabis products outside of work

- New York

  New York City bans pre-employment screening for marijuana use except for safety and security sensitive jobs and jobs bound by a federal or state contract or grant

There is a growing state by state pushback on pre employment testing. This is concerning because it seriously encroaches on the rights of the employer by removing their right to a sober workforce. It wouldn't be this way if there was a test that could determine impairment, but since there is not and all of these pre employment screens are by urinalysis, we are back to the issue in our scenario with Chris and me.

There are plenty of ways to go about employment related screening more thoughtfully. A couple of years ago we hired a therapist who tested positive for THC on their pre-employment test for the treatment center where I work. This may at first sound like a contradiction but there were important factors to be weighed. This individual was not in recovery so it was not critical to their employment. HR sat down with the candidate and explained the dilemma with testing and asked what was going on. The individual explained how they had been on vacation in a legal state prior to applying for this job. While they were there, they smoked some weed. Rather than probe too much, HR explained that with limited use like that it would be pretty hard to imagine having a positive test about a month post use. HR then asked the employee what date they would like to retest and they agreed on a month after the time they smoked weed on their vacation. Betting on the honesty of the employee, HR had them start the job training, which takes a ton of time, and attend meetings just not do anything directly with patients. At the end of 30 days they tested again and passed, the provisional offer became permanent and that was all there was to it.

But this scenario could have gone another way if the potential employee said they used weed responsibly outside of work hours and intended to continue using. At that point we would have rescinded the offer, because we need to be able to guarantee a sober workforce, and parted ways on friendly terms. If they wanted to use THC more than they wanted to work for us, who are we to force anything? This same thinking should apply the other way around. If it is more important to the employer to guarantee a sober employee than to hire the individual, the employer should have that right. Unfortunately, laws governing the workplace, like those we are starting to see passed in some states, take away that choice from the employer.

Let me be very clear; I do not have an issue with an adult using THC outside of work hours. This is not about judging any individual and their personal choices, but it is about safety and employer rights. I was once told in a debate that I advocated for determining a person's worth by their urine lab results. This is not about worth or ability to do a job when sober. This is about the poor state of testing for THC, the need for that to improve quickly and dramatically, and, until that happens, the only logical solution and the only way to prove sobriety in the workplace is zero measurable THC in a person's system.

One last thought, if using THC is more important than keeping or getting a job you might want to take a hard look at your use. In the addiction chapter, there are eleven diagnostic criteria for determining if a person has a substance use disorder and how severe it is. Two of those criteria are: "Not managing to do what you should at work, home or school, because of substance use" and "Giving up important social, occupational or recreational activities because of substance use". Both of those criteria would be met by choosing to use rather than being employed.

A while back I was involved in the treatment of a professional athlete who was addicted to both alcohol and THC. Part of the agreement with the team/league was that if he failed to complete 30 days in treatment he would be released and would forfeit more money than I will see in my lifetime. Two weeks into treatment, it got to be more than he could handle and he started packing up to leave. As I sat on his bed pulling clothing out of the suitcase he was packing and trying to reach him, I reminded him of this provision in his agreement and not only how much money he was walking away from but that his career may never bounce back. He was kind, as always, and thanked me for my concern but told me he just had to go and that he was never going to use again (the scariest thing a departing patient can say) and that he would be just fine. As he walked out the front door and jumped in a waiting car one of my coworkers pointed out the money he was loosing and said, "What a dumbass." I quickly corrected them with, "What a perfect example of addiction and powerlessness." If getting high is more important than working, it may be more than foolishness, it may be a symptom of addiction; consider calling someone for help.

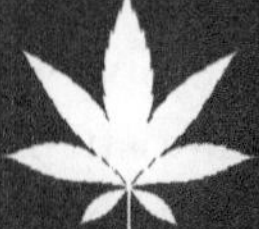

CHAPTER

07

"WHAT CAN'T THEY DO?"

The industry knows no limits on it's products

We built the pyramids. We put a man on the moon. We sequenced the human genome. And now, thanks to human ingenuity and technological prowess, we have weed water! That's right, there are now multiple companies selling THC infused water

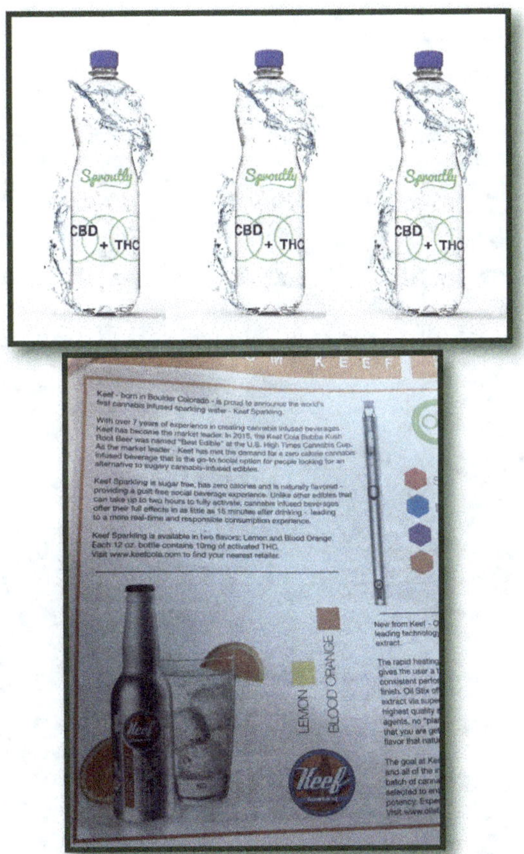

There was a story in The Denver Post 6/24/16, now ancient history, with a humdinger of a title, "Infused Everything: These Cannabis Products Might Surprise You:[1] Coffee, Post-tattoo ointment, toothpaste, vaginal suppositories; the staggering variety begs the question, 'What can't we infuse?'"

Infused everything: These cannabis products might surprise you

Coffee. Post-tattoo ointment. Toothpaste. Um, vaginal suppositories? The staggering variety begs the question, 'What can't we infuse?'

PUBLISHED: JUN 24, 2016, 7:27 PM • UPDATED: 7 DAYS AGO

ADD A COMMENT

By **Katie Shapiro**, *The Cannabist Staff*

Move over edibles, lotions and tincture potions — there's an entire new realm of cannabis-infused products hitting the shelves of dispensaries and recreational shops as marijuana moves even further into the mainstream.

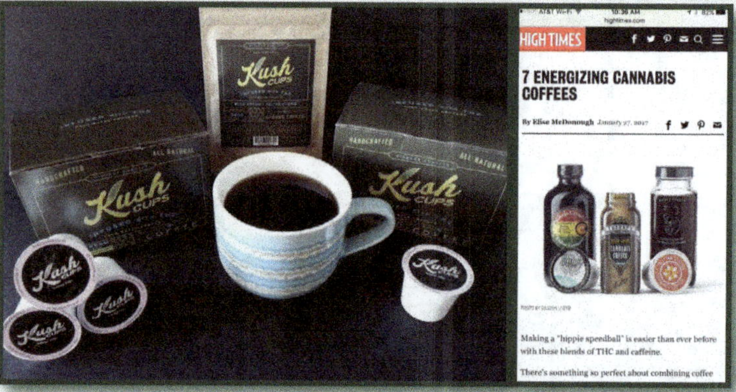

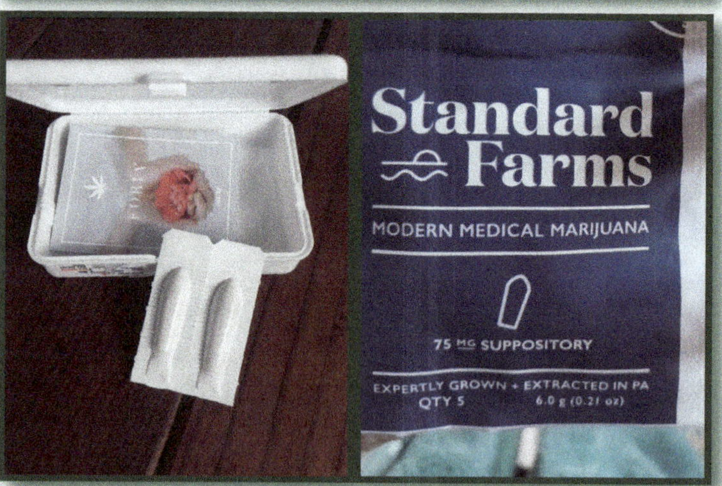

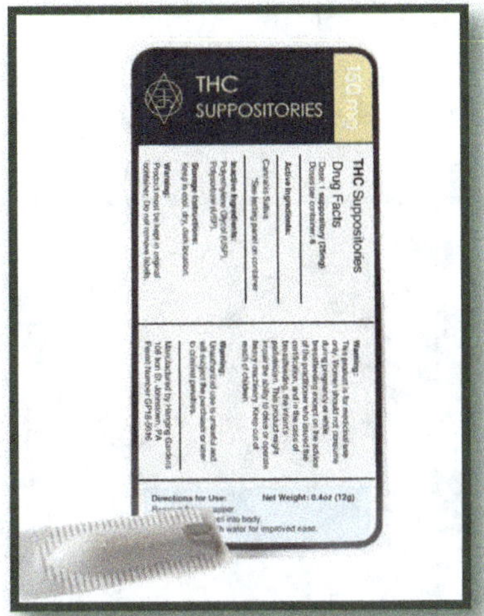

Apparently, the answer is "nothing"! If it can be introduced into the human body, someone is infusing it with THC and selling it, often with kids in mind. This is an issue for a number of reasons, the most obvious concerns how easy these products are to conceal and use in plain sight. Think of kids in school; few administrators are looking for the THC infused lollipops, pictured below..

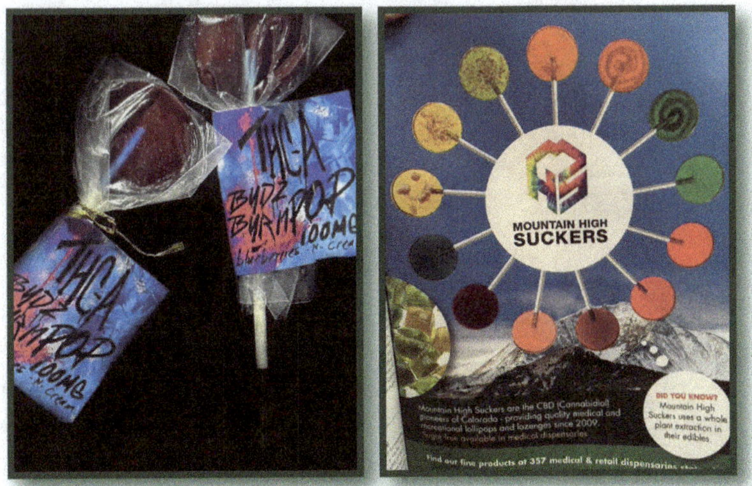

The other big issue is that we are putting a ton of hope in oral testing procedures. Those tests won't pick up the intoxicating THC deodorant or topical THC cream. In addition, there are many products being made that are, despite claims to the contrary, intended to appeal to kids. Seriously, how many adults are buying "Pot Rocks,"

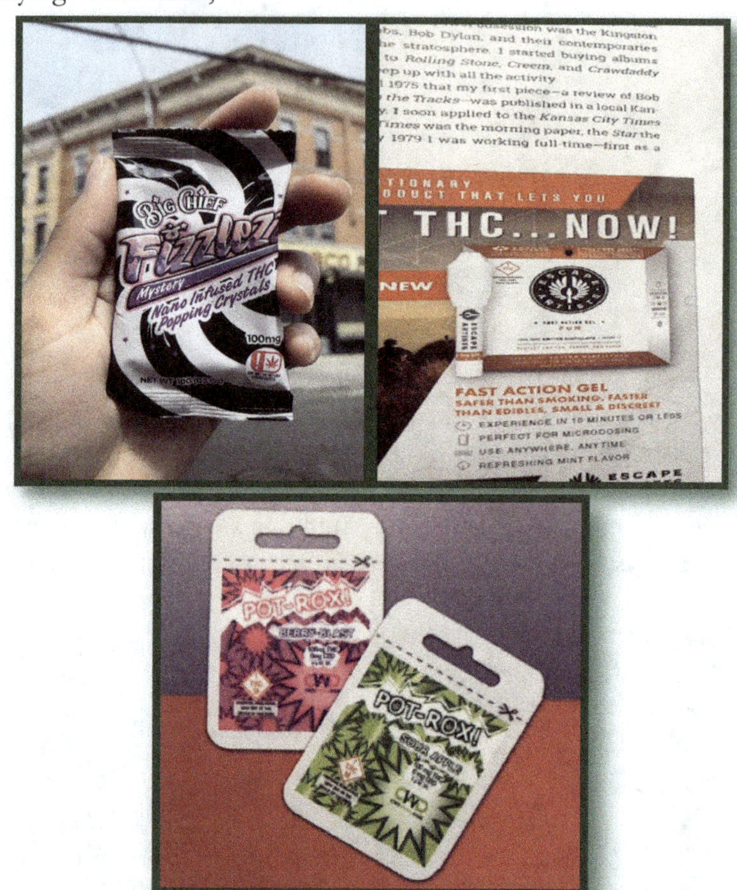

a THC-infused popping candy made to look like pop rocks? There are also products with the specific intent of capturing more of the minority market, like THC syrup.

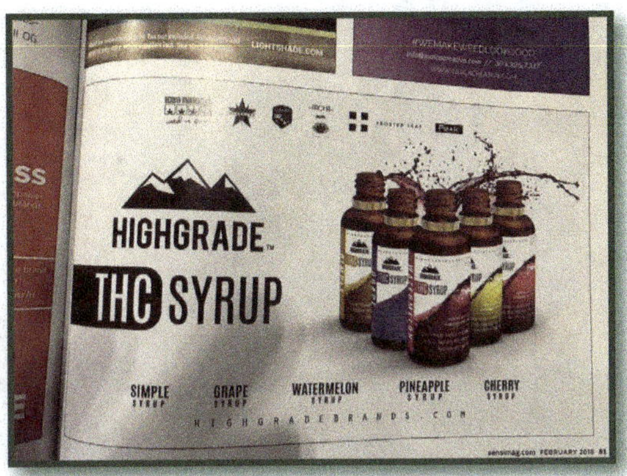

I guess that one could also apply to Post Malone and Macilm-ore and they are white, but I digress. The last big issue I want to point out is that many of these products and the means by which they are ingested or introduced into the human body are untested in any reliable scientific way. As an example, a couple of years ago a filmmaker named Jane Wells came to Colorado to work on a documentary that would ultimately be called "Pot-Luck." She somehow got my number and we met up to talk about THC. Part of the discussion dealt with how easy it is for the Indus-try to bypass and outmaneuver the regulatory system. Case in point: accepting credit cards to pay for THC products, which is a way of legally laundering drug money by integrating it into the mainstream financial market. Jane was having a hard time believ-ing THC could be openly purchased with a credit card, because it is illegal to use credit cards! We were in downtown Boulder and I told Jane to pick any store she wanted. I would go in and buy THC with a credit card (so long as she paid me back). She picked a store, I walked in and started browsing. The first thing that caught my eye was a THC-infused candy bar. I grabbed it and headed towards the check out.

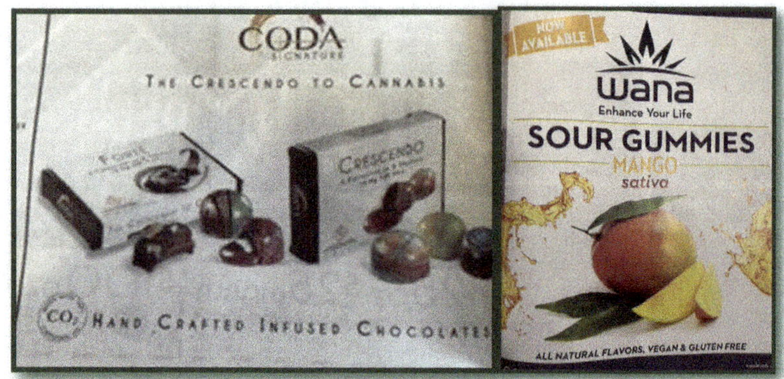

As I approached the counter, I noticed a THC suppository for sale; I asked for one of those as well. As the budtender was ringing up my credit card sale, I noticed that the suppositories had 70mg's of THC in each and I was buying a pack of two. Knowing that the legal limit per serving was then and still is 10mg, I asked the young lady how someone is expected to consume 1/7th of a suppository. She gave me a blank look so I continued; "Do I insert it REALLY REALLY slowly over the course of a day or two? Or should I break it off into 7ths and shove that up my ass?" She laughed a little bit at the obvious rookie buying this product and told me to take the whole thing at once. I feigned surprise, "Seven legal servings at once, isn't that bad?" She smiled and told me that it would be "an awesome high." Using my credit card to buy highly concentrated THC, intended to be used via a fast-delivery system, I was specifically told to take 7 'legal' doses at once! This is a small glimpse into the realities of Colorado's "tightly regulated market."

When people are introduced to pictures of all the "edibles" that can be purchased, they are shocked. The breadth of THC-infused products is astonishing. For the last few years I've offered to buy dinner for anyone that can find something consumable that is not for sale with THC in it. So far, I've been dining alone!

Before browsing through some revealing pictures, I want to point out what I think is the biggest oversight in the law on this subject. It's not the fact that you can buy one package with one clear serving, like this cake pop

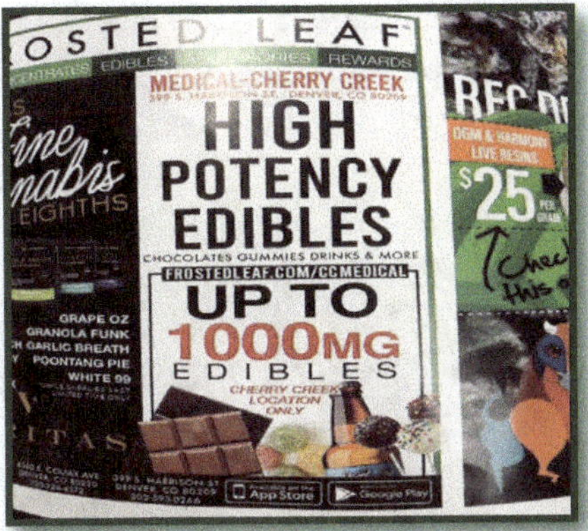

with 1000mg's or 100 legal servings. The biggest issue is that we continue to measure servings based on dry weight of the cannabis plant when in reality things are being infused with everything but the flower. They're using distillates!

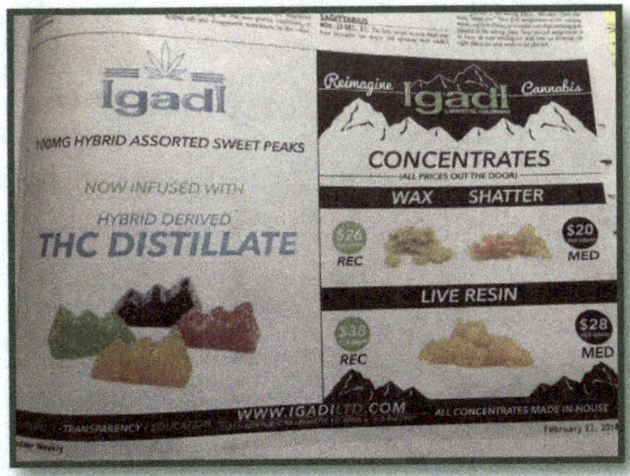

Let me lay out the complex math to convert 10mg of flower in an edible to 10mg of concentrates in an edible: $n-x2(\%+52.7)$ = Nevermind, I have no idea how to do that conversion and neither does anyone else. Rather than regulating edibles by weight, it should be based upon potency. Until this issue is addressed you will have the industry providing pseudo-science to consumers. For instance, there is a handy chart (available for 21 year olds and up) on Leafly.com. (Remember, the legal limit per serving is 10mg

THC.) This chart is intended to help the user determine if they should take a 2.5mg dose or a 1000mg dose![2] The insanity of the THC-infused edibles market is real, scary, and in plain view. While you browse the pictures, imagine the kids who are browsing and using the products!

Baked goods

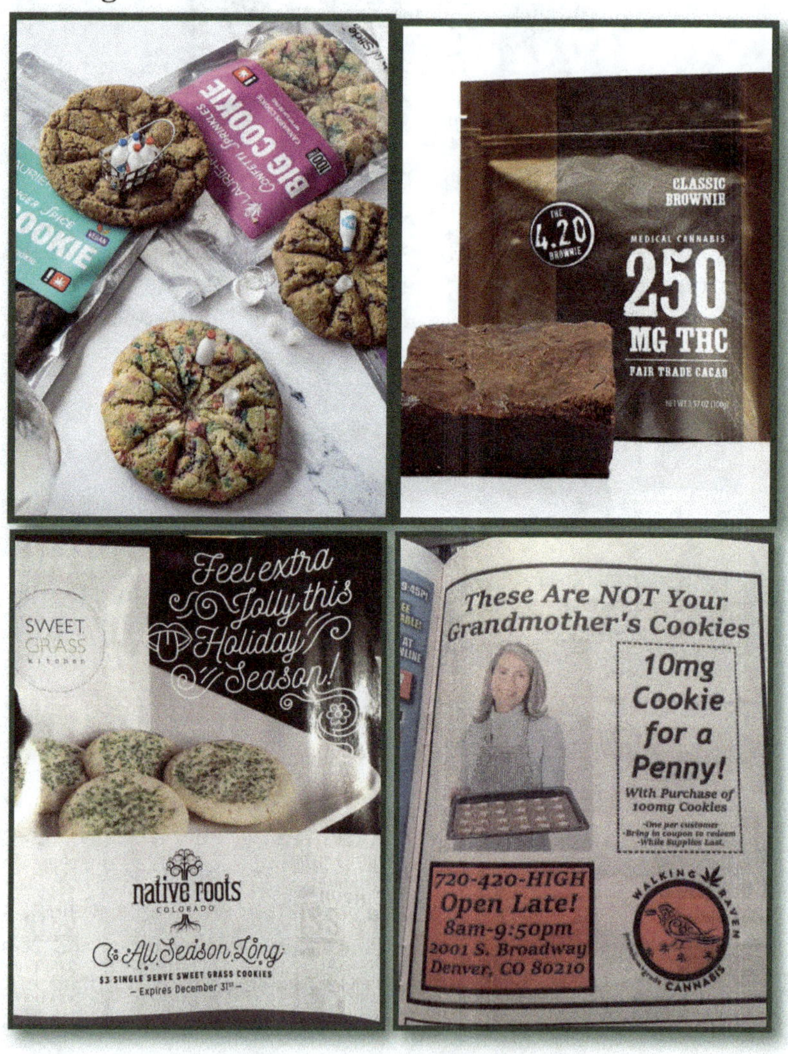

Candy bars

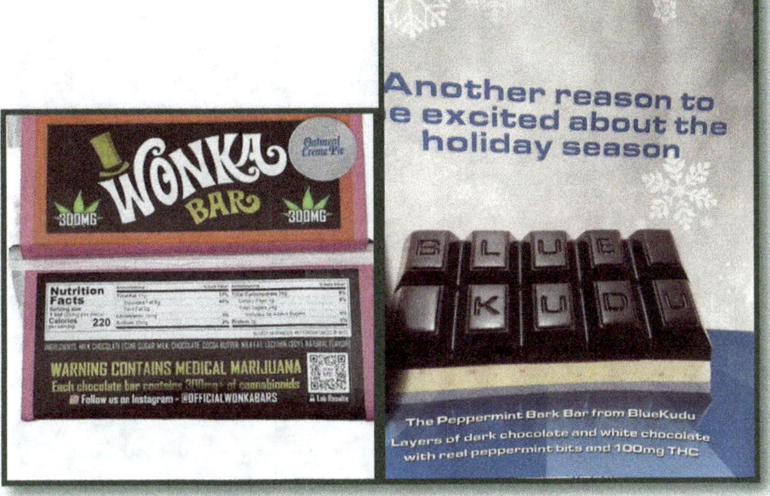

Granola bars

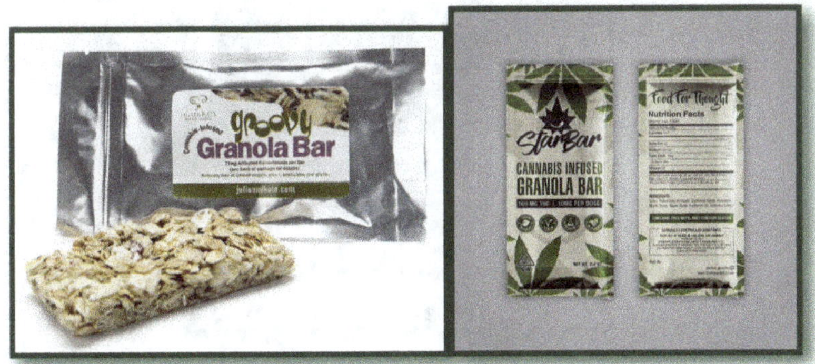

Ice cream

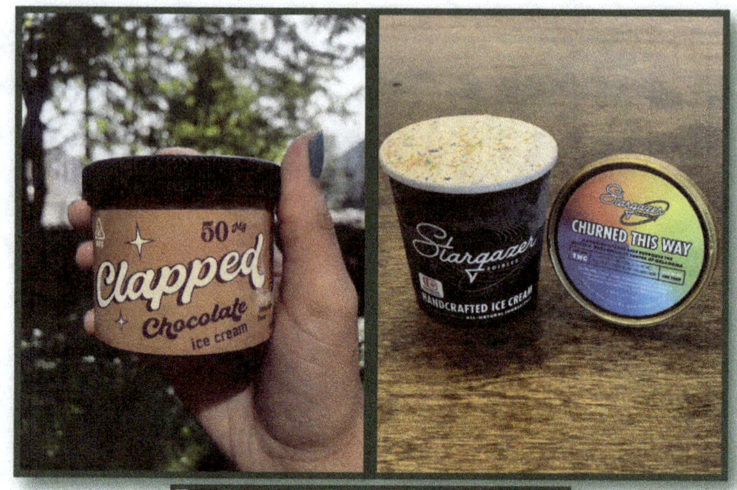

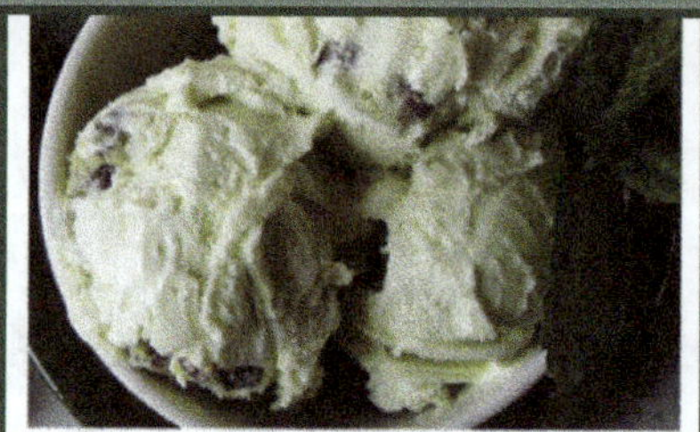

Marijuana Infused Ice Cream

Embark on a never ending munchies loop as you indulge in a sweet bowl of marijuana infused ice cream. This sugary treat comes laced with grade-A funk that'll leave you feeling like your brain and body have melted into a carefree nirvana.

$15.00

Hard candies

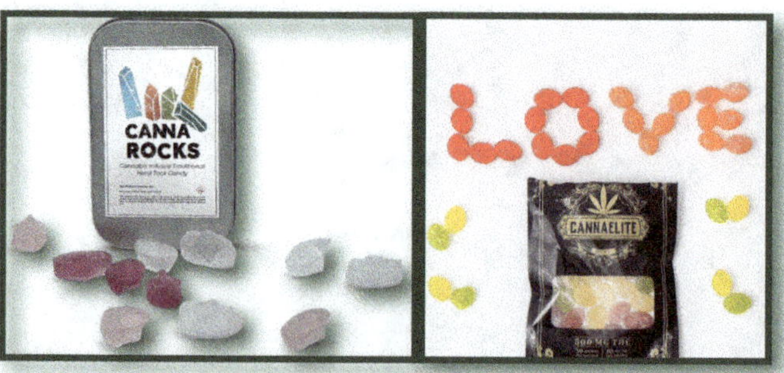

Soft candies

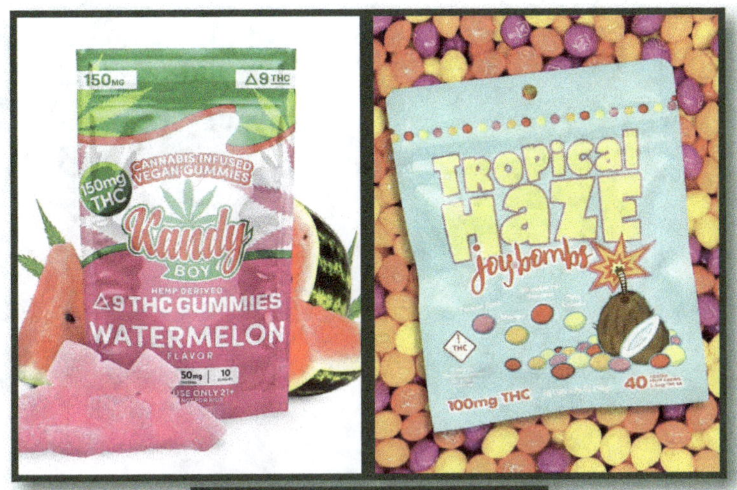

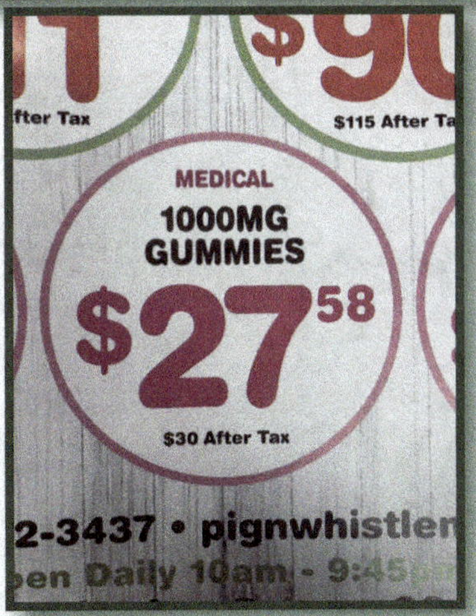

Gummy bears/worms/drops

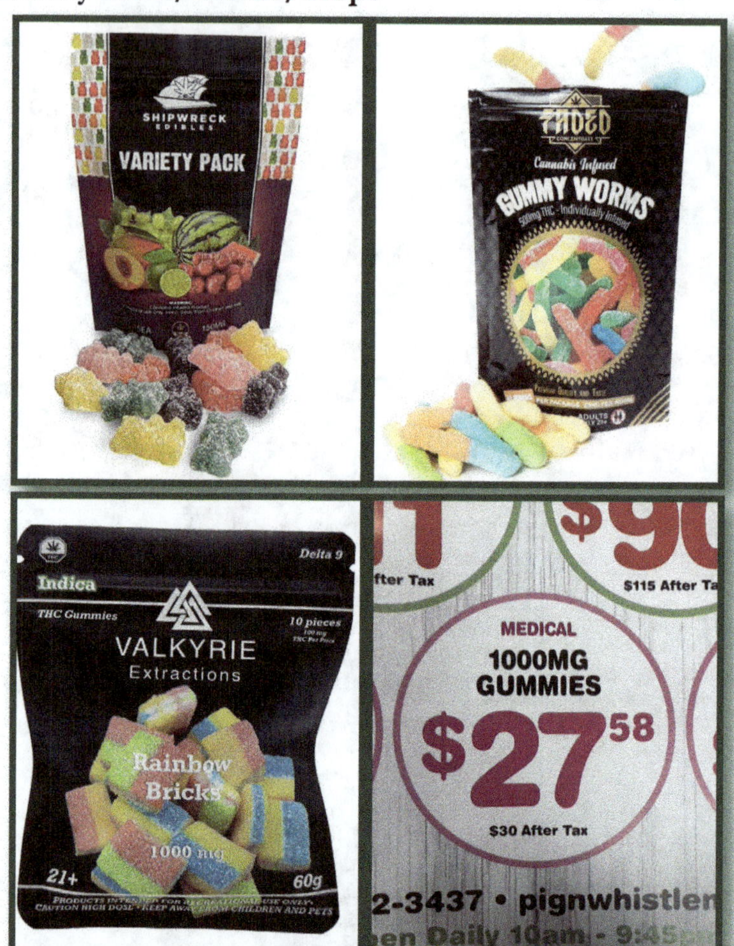

Hot sauce

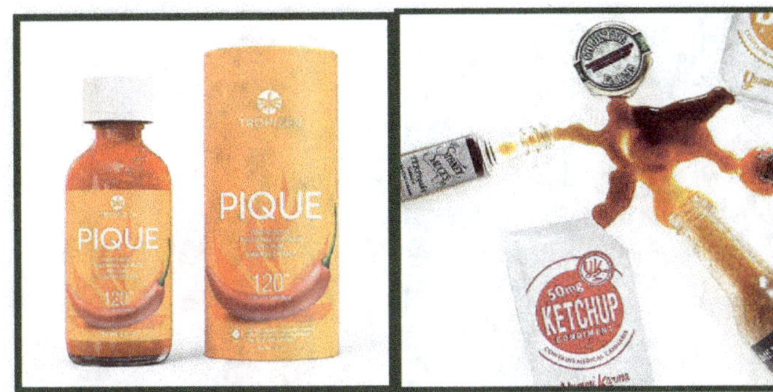

Ketchup

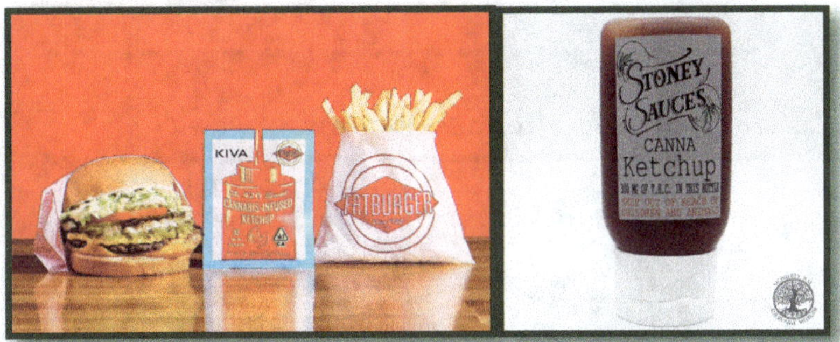

Mustard

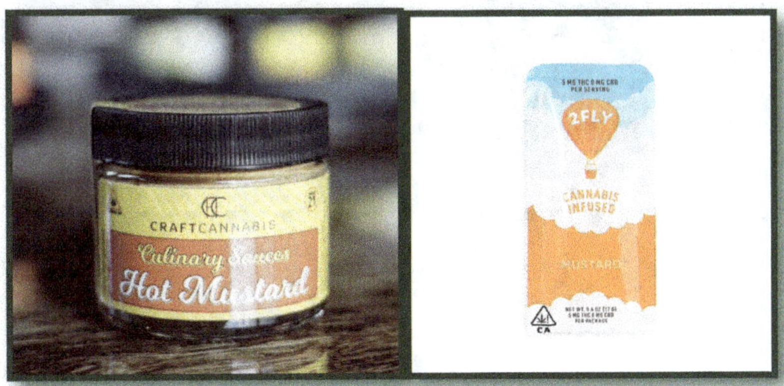

BBQ sauce

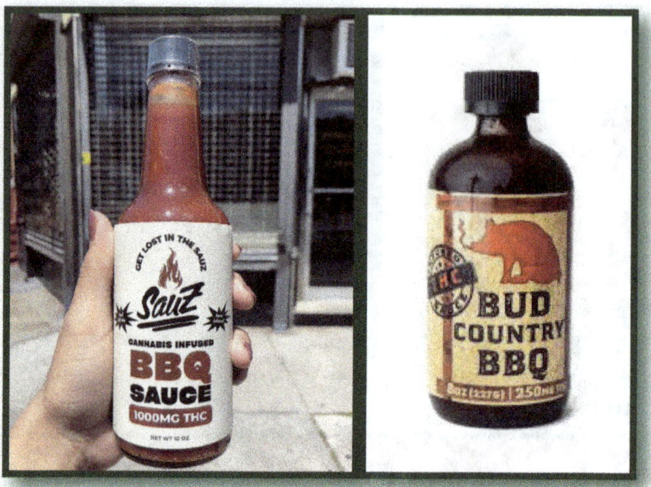

Coffee (cold brew, grounds, k-cup)

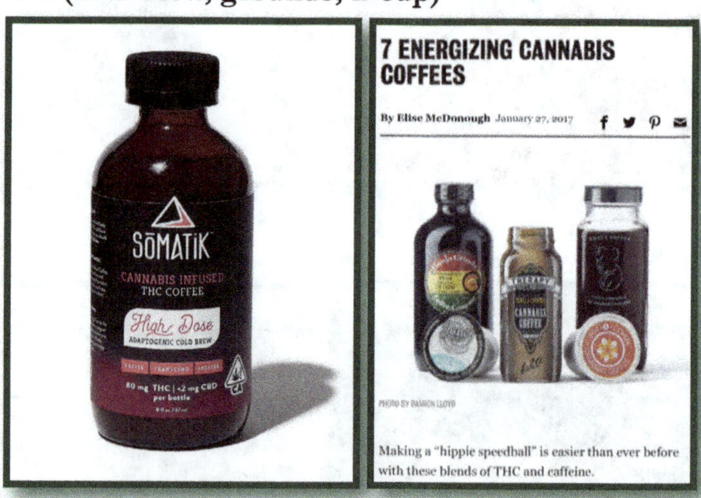

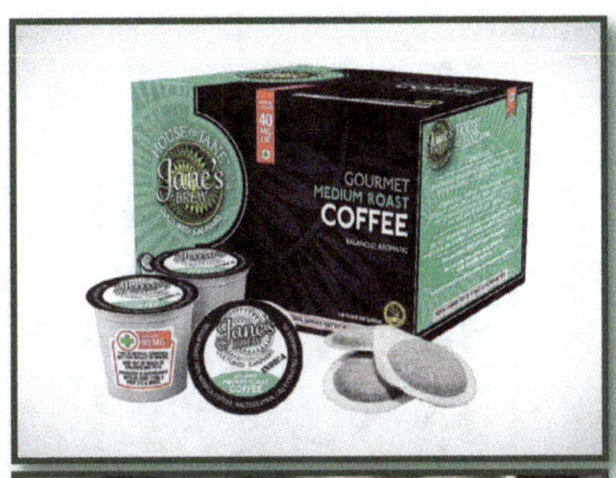

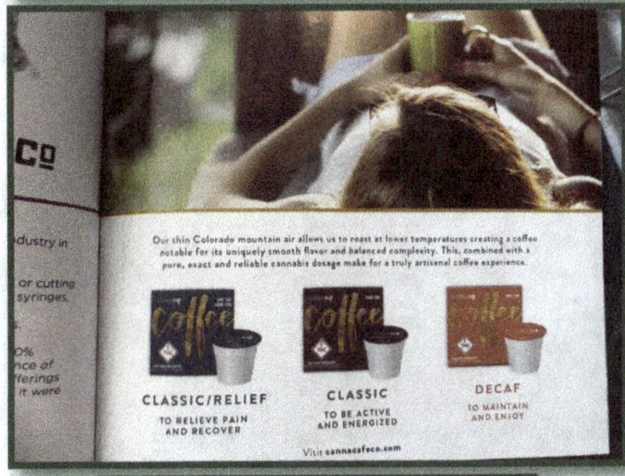
Our thin Colorado mountain air allows us to roast at lower temperatures creating a coffee notable for its uniquely smooth flavor and balanced complexity. This, combined with a pure, exact and reliable cannabis dosage make for a truly artisenal coffee experience.
CLASSIC/RELIEF
TO RELIEVE PAIN AND RECOVER
CLASSIC
TO BE ACTIVE AND ENERGIZED
DECAF
TO MAINTAIN AND ENJOY
Visit cannacafeco.com

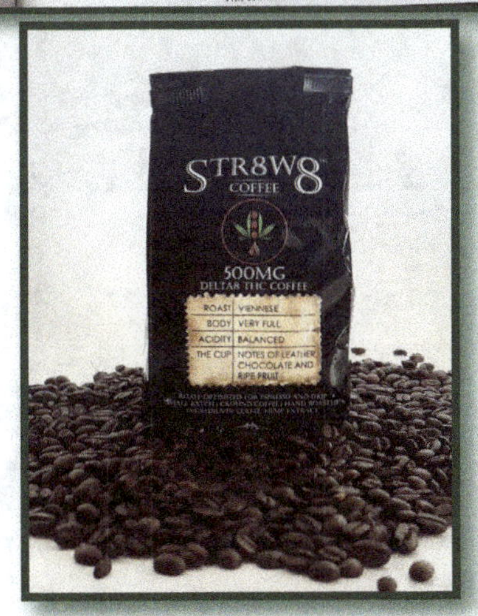
STR8W8
COFFEE
500MG
DELTA8 THC COFFEE
ROAST   VIENNESE
BODY   VERY FULL
ACIDITY   BALANCED
THE CUP   NOTES OF LEATHER, CHOCOLATE AND RIPE FRUIT

Topical ointment

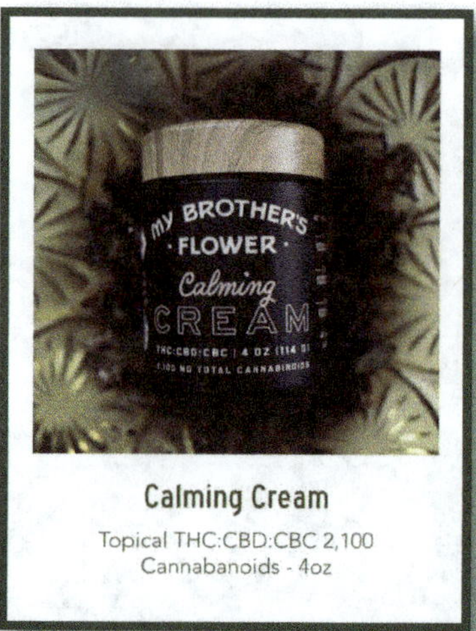

Calming Cream

Topical THC:CBD:CBC 2,100
Cannabanoids - 4oz

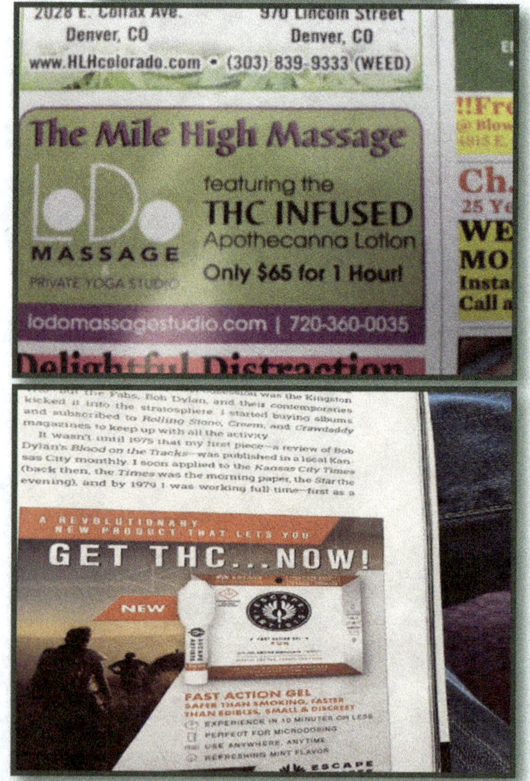

Swallowable pills (available in both indica and sativa)

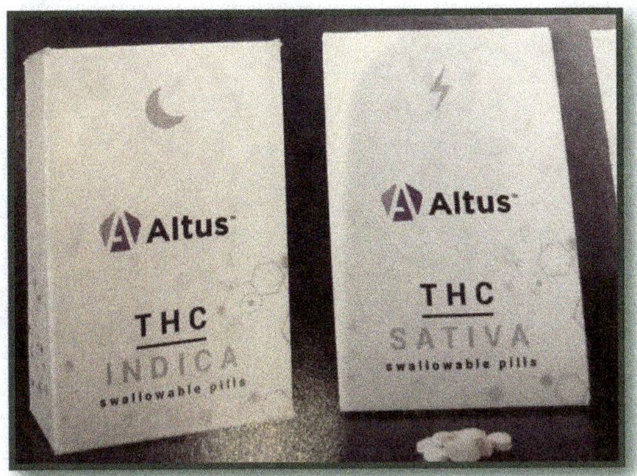

Lollipops

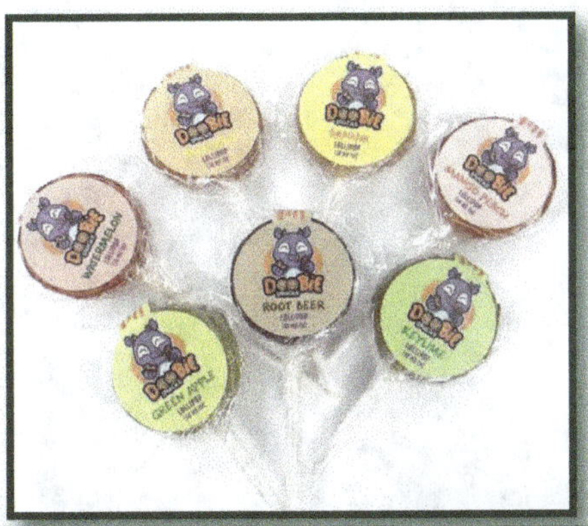

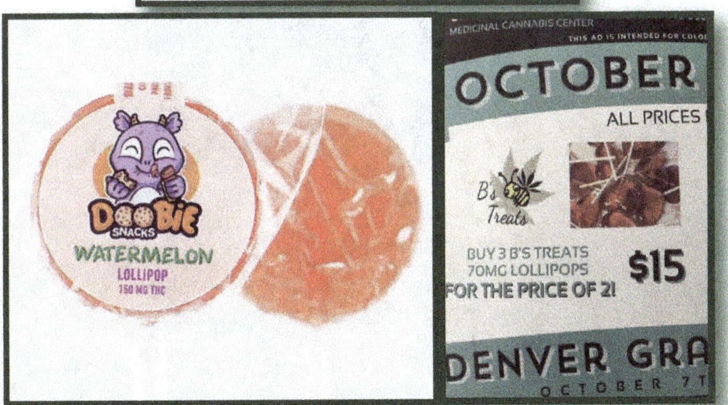

Tea

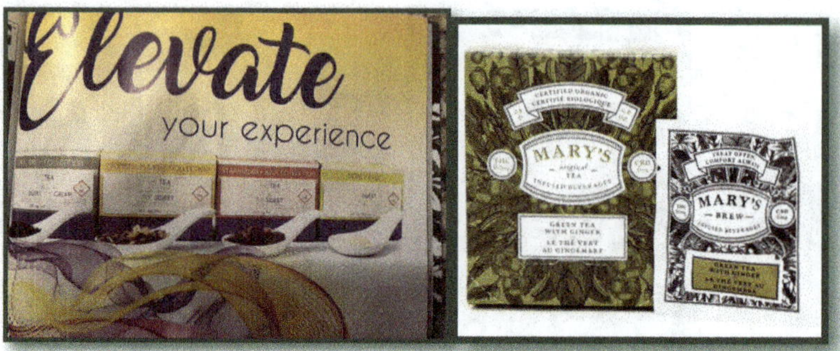

Soda

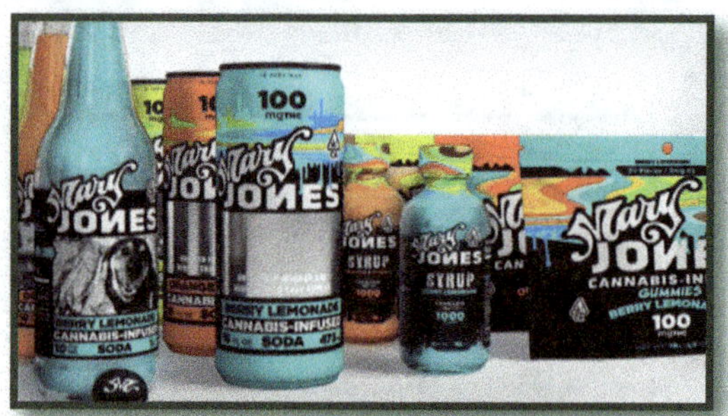

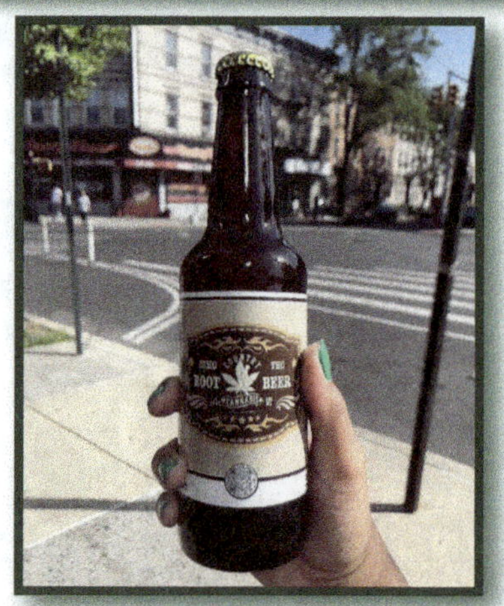

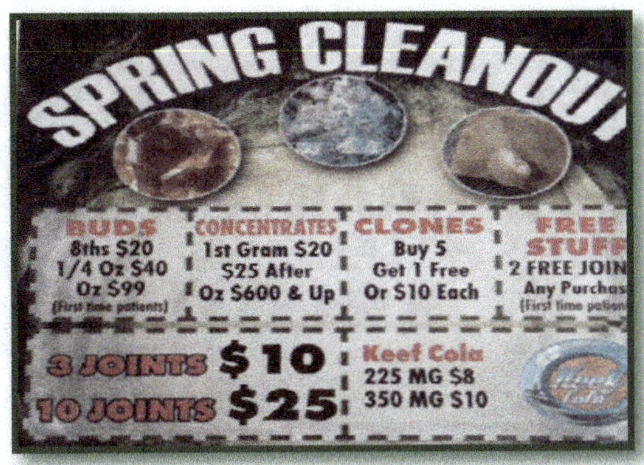

Water (of course)

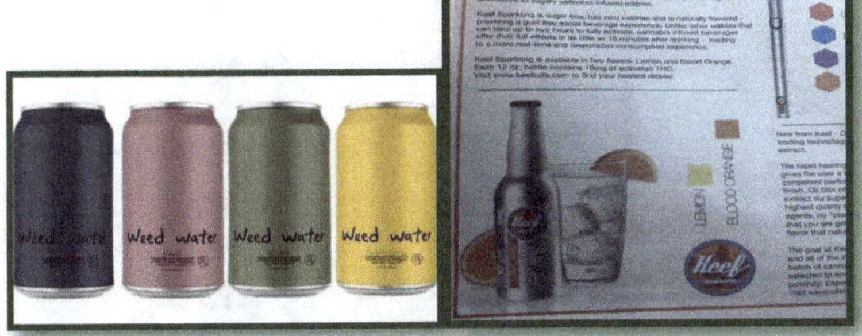

Juice

SUNRISE
CANNABIS
CANNABIS
INFUSED
JUICE
TROPICAL PUNCH
1000MG THC
9:04 AM
wm
Pure & Simple
0.0 RATING
+ FOLLOW
PRODUCTS   NEAR ME   REVIEWS   VIDEOS   INST
Beverages
VIEW ALL
Assorted Juice
Blend 100mg
0.0
Hibiscus Citrus
Juice Blend 100...
0.0
Minty Lime
Blend 100m
0.0

ROOT
BEER
FRUIT
PUNCH
BERRY
LEMONADE
CHERRY
LIMEADE
HALF
& HALF
100
100
100
100
100
MENTION THIS AD FOR
$4.20 OFF
ANY DIXIE PRODUCT

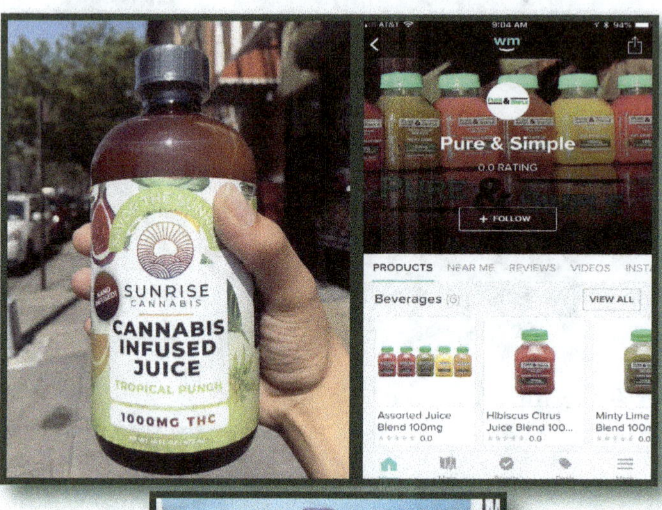

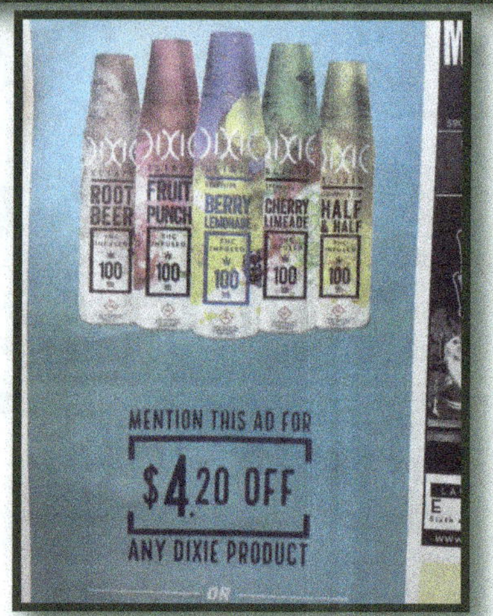

Chi Tea

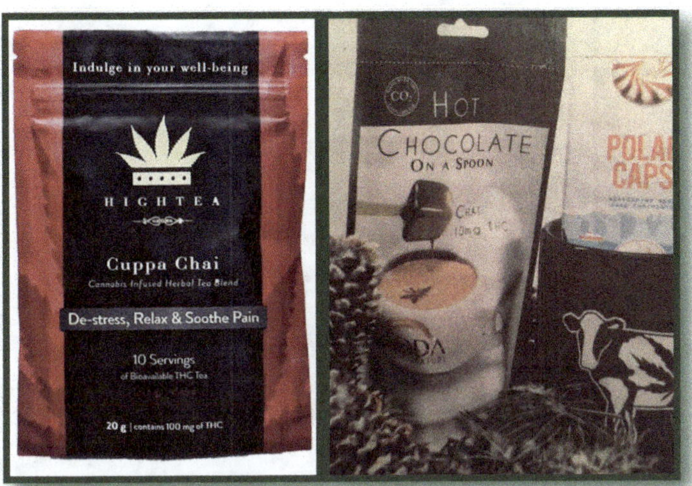

Mints

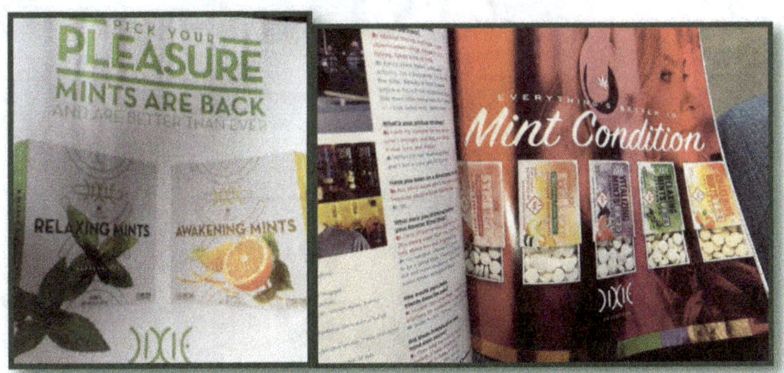

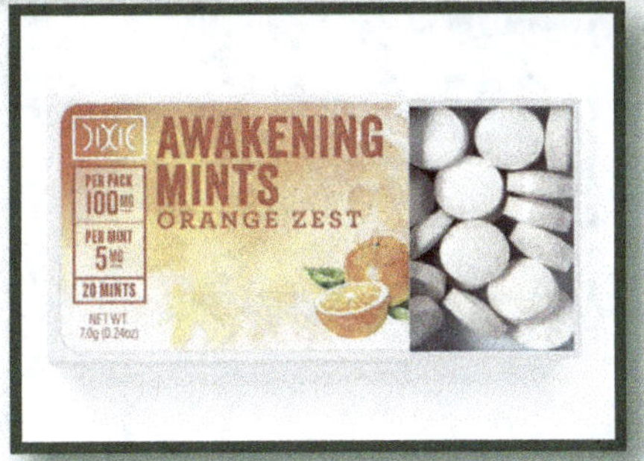

Breath spray

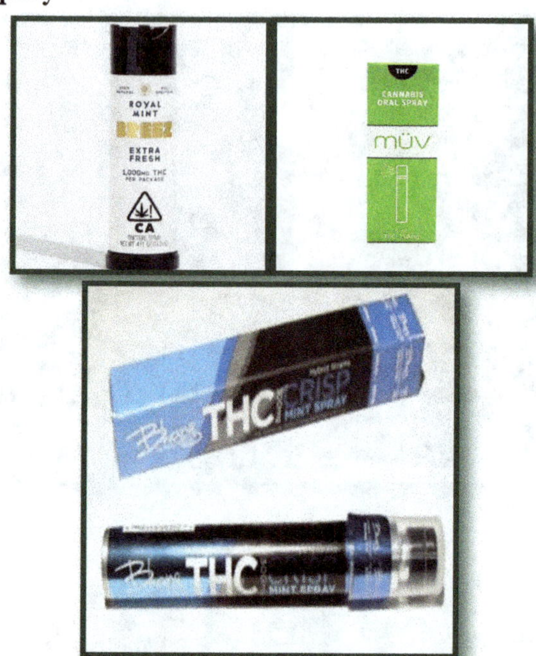

Wipes

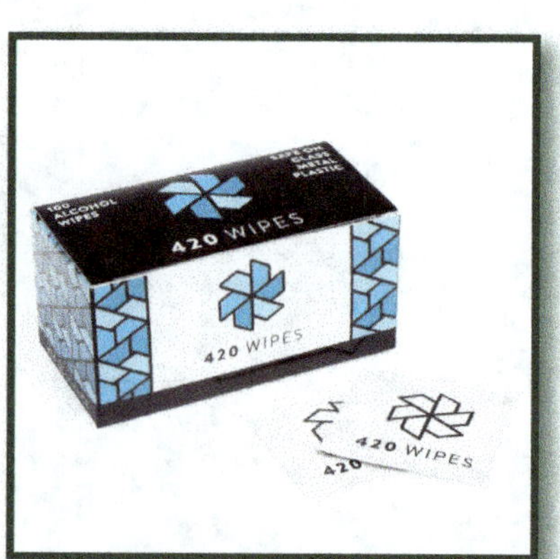

Potato chips

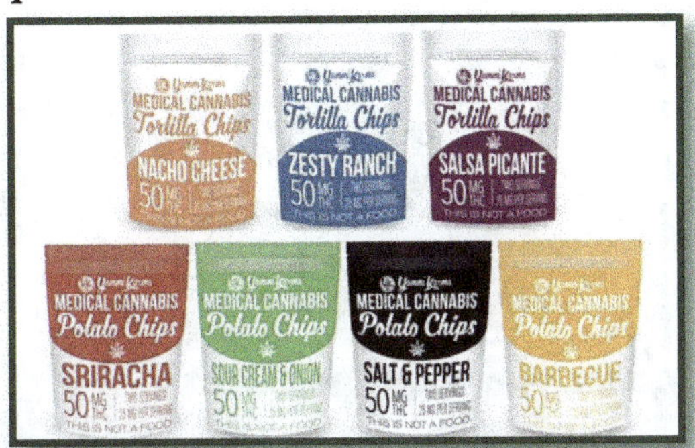

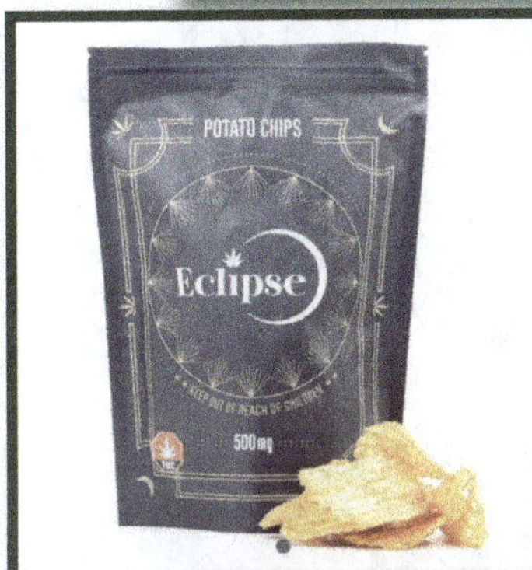

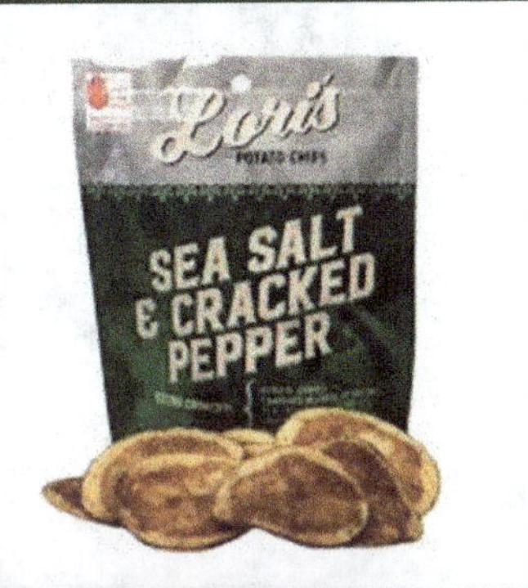

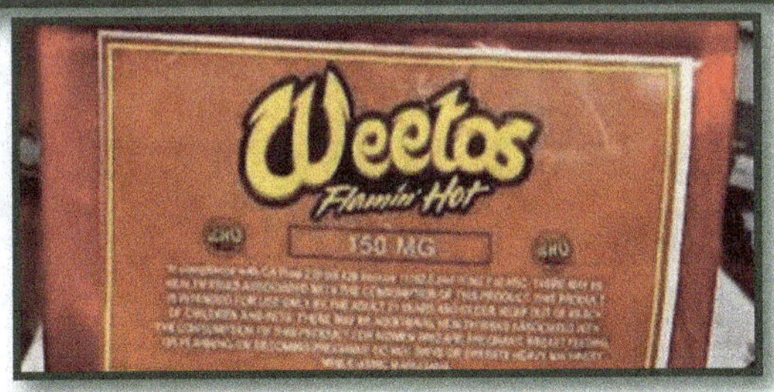

Tampons

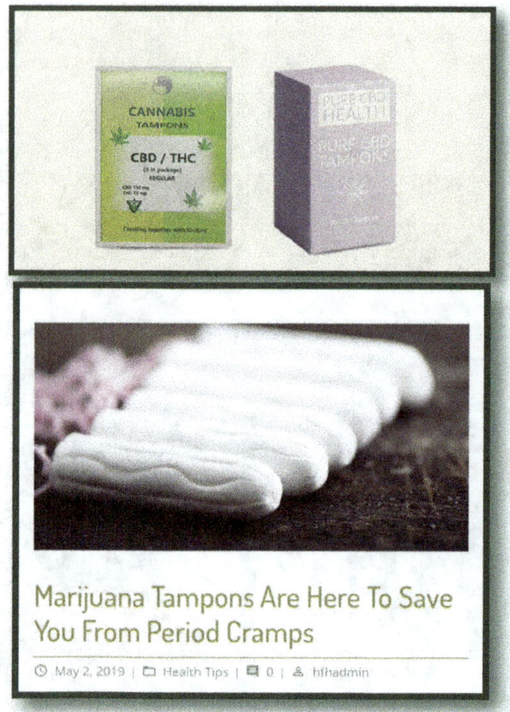

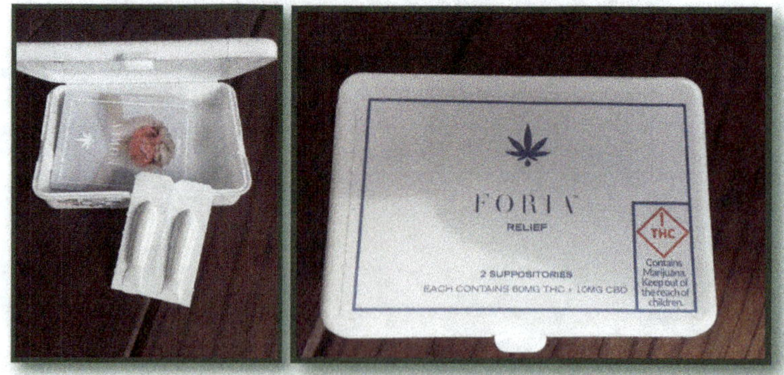

Suppositories

Gum

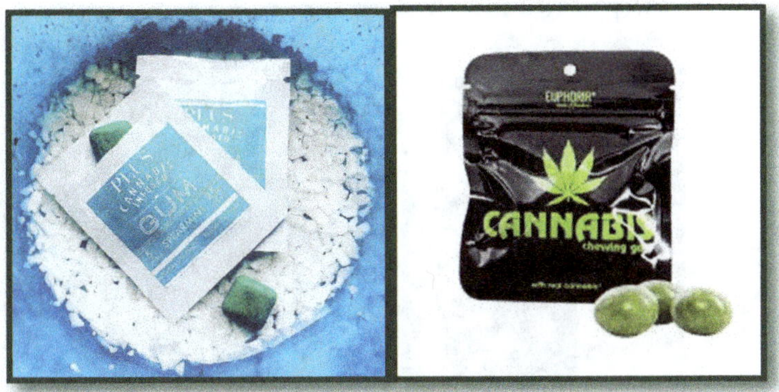

Liquid THC

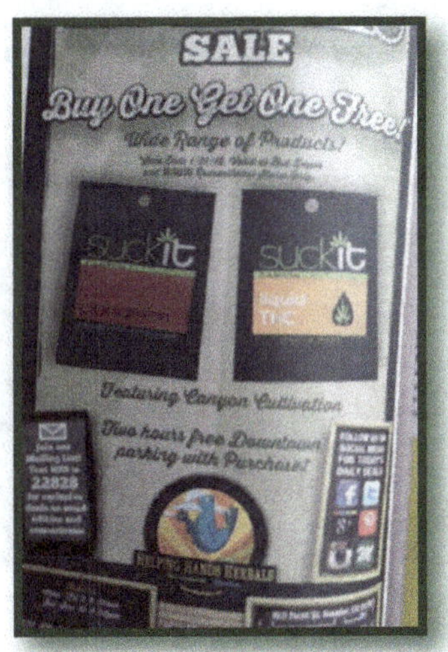

Five hour energy

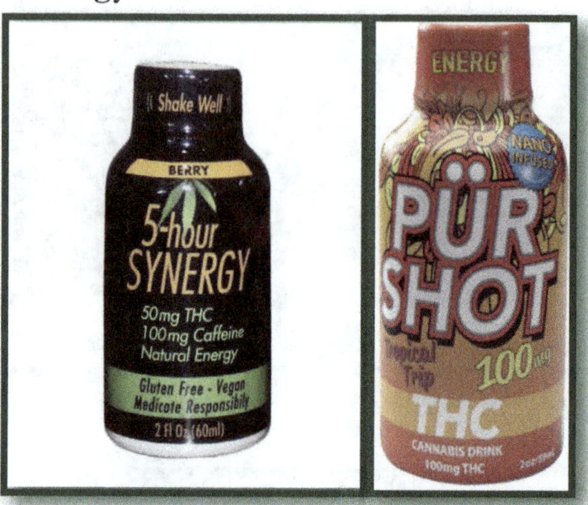

Deodorant

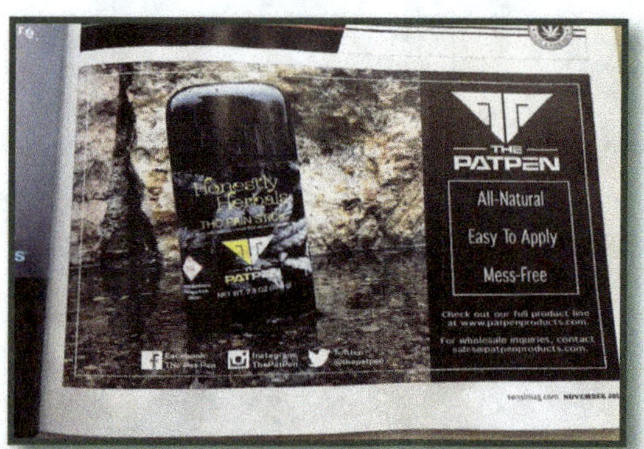

Sex Lube

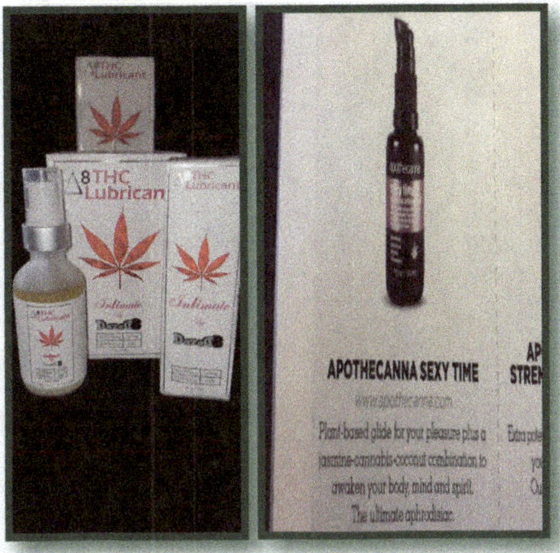

Taffy

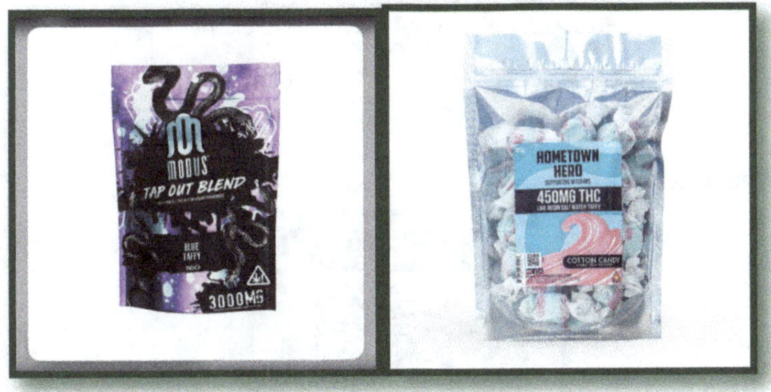

Pizza

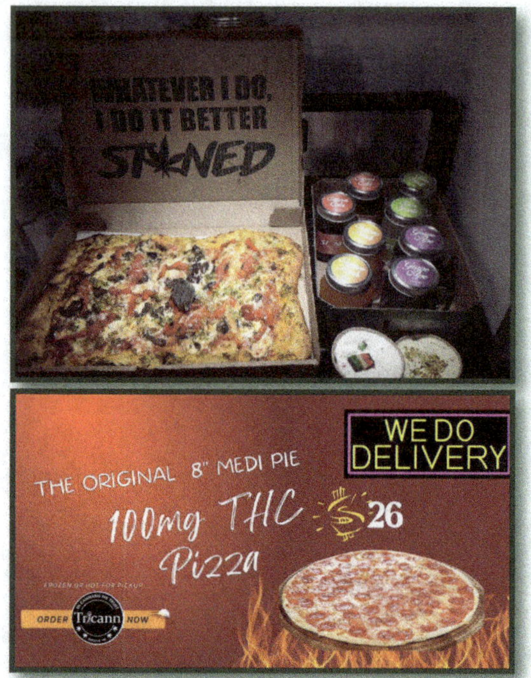

Spaghetti sauce

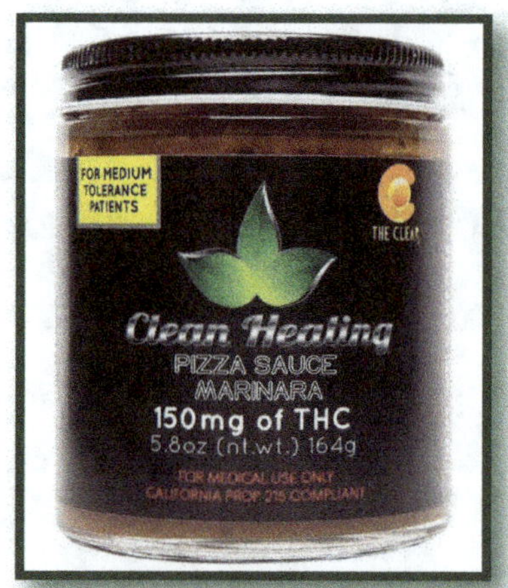

Cake

Ice Cream
Cakes
Locally Owned and Operated
1146
1144
MUST BE 18
&
HAVE
ID READY
OPEN
Product details
Strawberry Vanilla Pound Cake
Bite, 10 servings of 10 MG
THC(100 MG THC Total)
Sold By: LHF
Sign Up to Shop
Log In
Product information
License
Category   Edibles & Ingestibles
Subcategory   Baked Goods (non-
                  cookie)
Classification   Hybrid
Product description
Made with real strawberries!
Previous product   Next product

Nuts

D9 NUTS
SWEET BOURBON
COMPLIANT
GROWN in TN

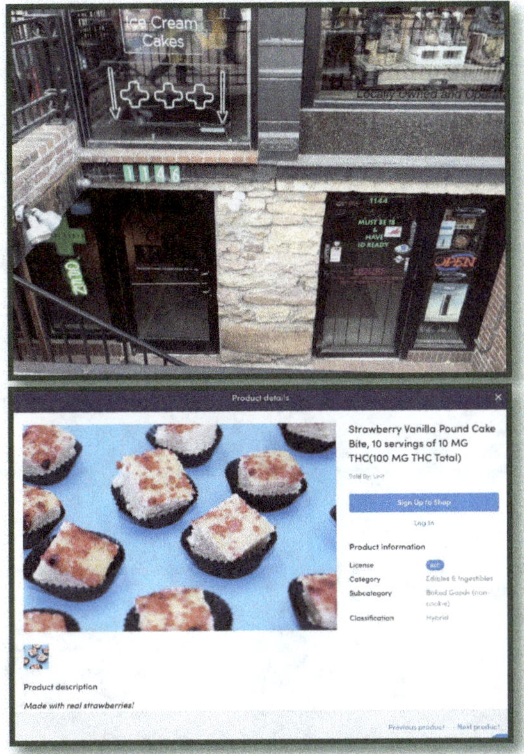

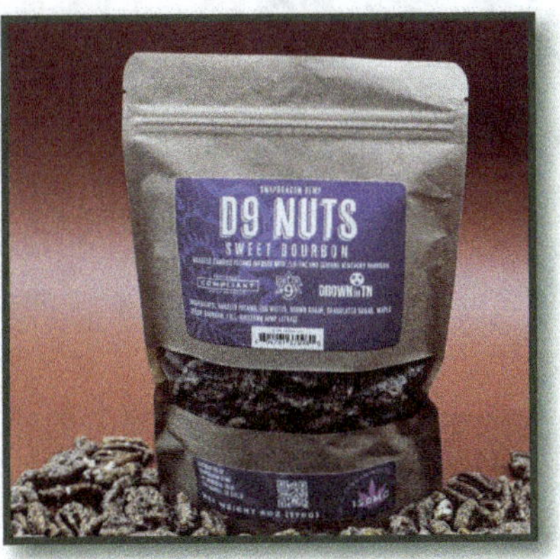

Popsicles

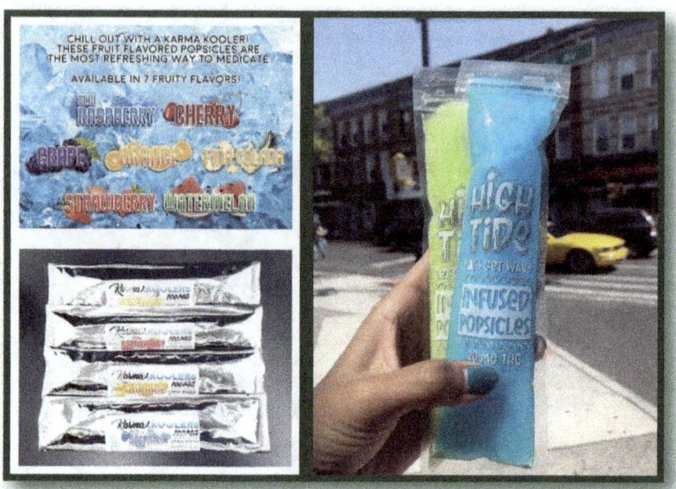

Goldfish

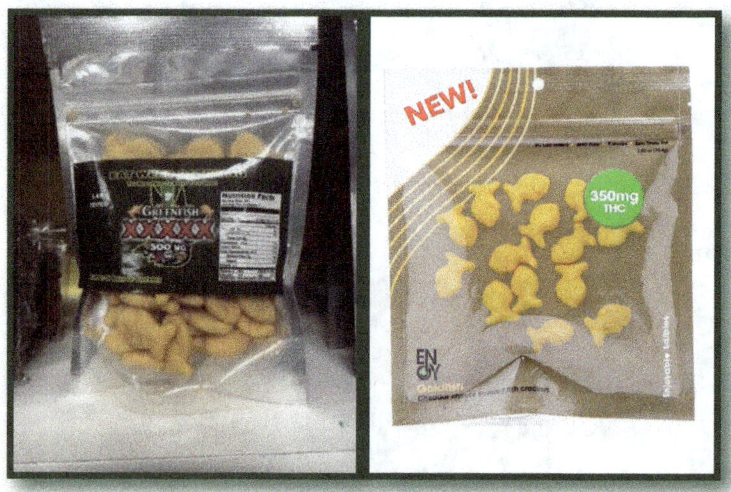

Pot rocks

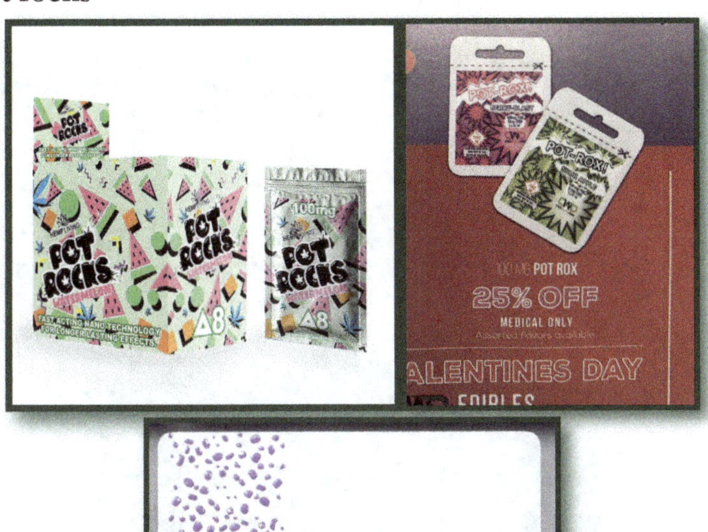

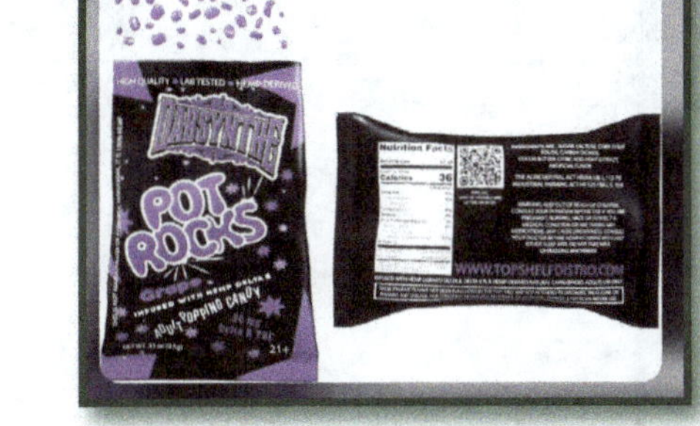

Honey

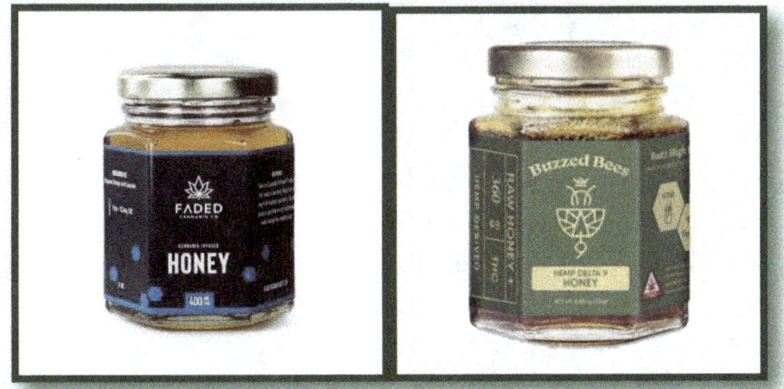

Jelly

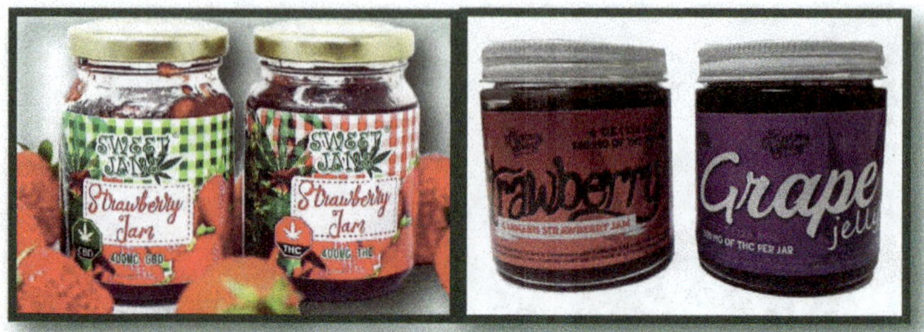

Transdermal Patches

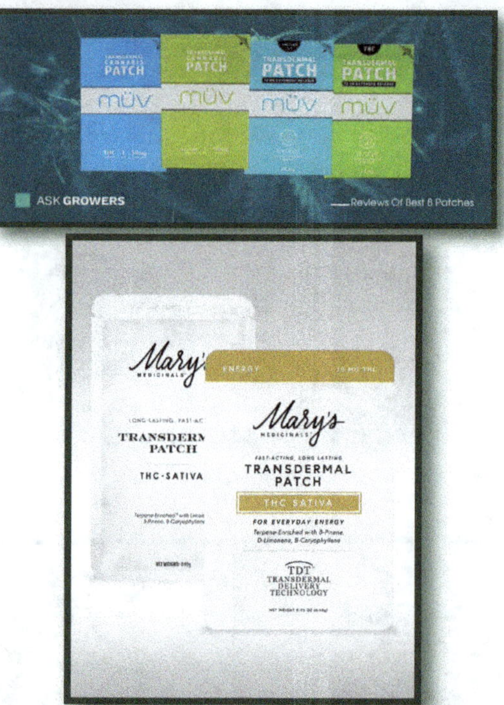

And of course Water soluble drops, with a bottle of this you can turn anything into an edible.

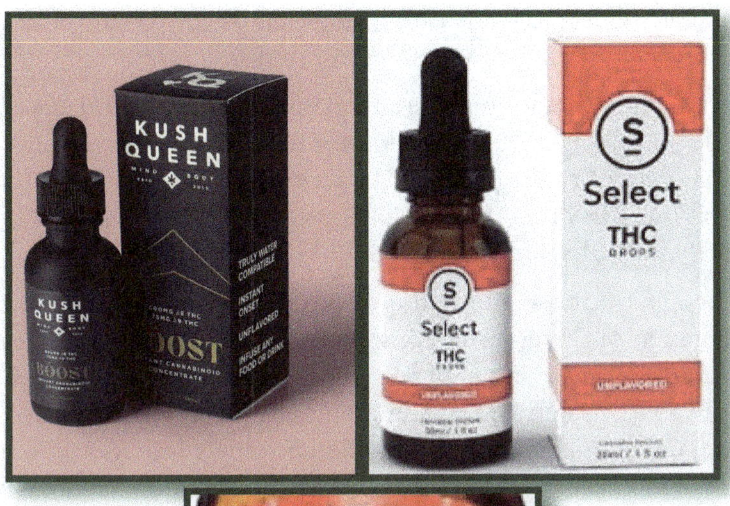

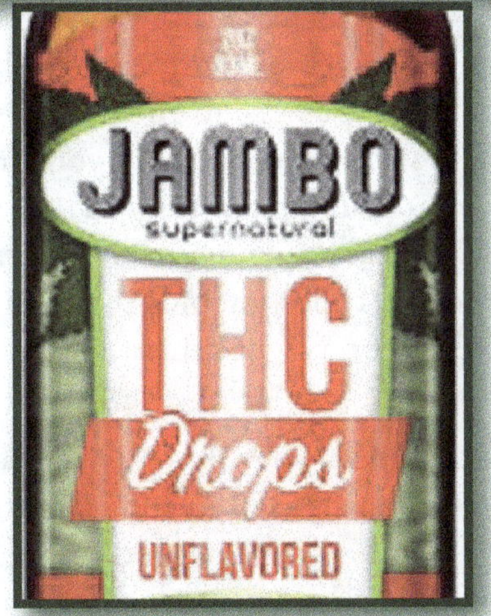

This is a serious issue because these drops make it possible for a person to open an ordinary can of soda (not infused), put a few drops in it, and, voila, it's infused with intoxicating THC. Think about it, you can sit down at family dinner, wait for your moment, put a few drops on the broccoli and boom! This stuff has also complicated things in the treatment world; imagine how it impacts searching patients entering treatment. The program where I work is voluntary, only people who want to be there are there. We deal with this challenge less than involuntary programs, but the real losers are the schools. I spent a few depressing hours watching videos of kids eating edibles in school. Sadly and unsurprisingly, it's not an uncommon practice.

"Overdose" is a noun meaning "an excessive and dangerous dose of a drug." ICD 10 codes are what medical providers use to bill for specific things. The ICD 10 code for "poisoning by cannabis" is T40.711D, and the billing code for intentionally doing self-harm with cannabis is T40.712A.

People overdose all the time from THC. Bearing in mind the definition of "overdose," consider the reality that most of those overdoses have edibles to blame. There are two kinds of OD from THC, intentional and unintentional and they are easy to define; intentional is when someone knowingly ingests too much and unintentional is when someone accidentally ingests too much.

The second scenario is easier to explain, think of being dosed. You walk into a friend's house, see a cup of coffee on the counter, and drink it. There's a terrified look on your friend's face when he walks in to see you draining the cup. "Dude, you just drank 30 servings of THC!" That's "unintentional." The much more likely real world scenario is a child grabbing a handful of THC candy or eating some baked goods while their caregivers are too stoned to notice.

"Intentional" is much more common. You walk into a friend's house and they offer you an infused gummy bear. Being a conscientious consumer you read the label and cut 1/10th of the gummy off, "one serving," and eat it, (remember, this is just pretend). Despite the label telling you that the effects may be delayed for up to two hours, you start to get a little concerned 20 minutes in because you're not feeling high. We are pretty accustomed to feeling the intoxicating effects of our drugs very quickly (drinking, smoking, snorting, shooting, etc.) and it has never taken this long when you smoked regular weed. You reexamine the label and there is the explanation: "this product was produced without regulatory oversight for health, safety or efficacy."

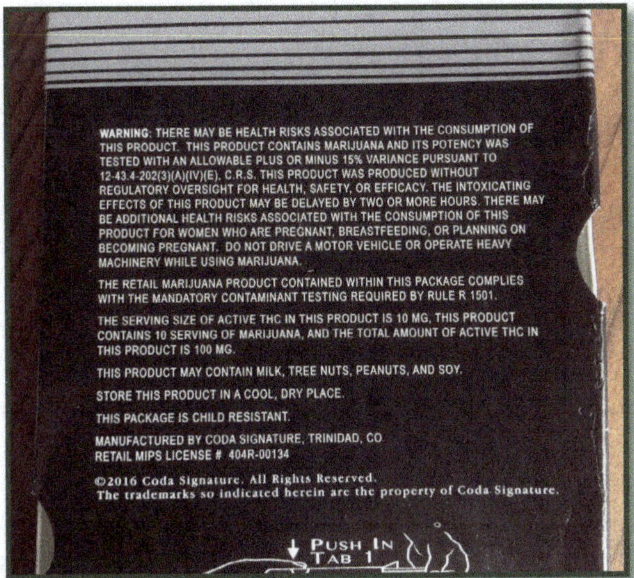

How did you miss that before! Since what you are eating has no quality controls in its production you figure that you must have eaten the ear of the gummy bear without THC, so you pop the rest of it in your mouth. Thirty minutes later, the effects of the 10 legal doses you just consumed start to kick in. Your blood pressure spikes, you get super anxious, then scared, then who knows what, depends on the person. Some people pass out, some get violent, some run into traffic, some hurt others, some jump out of the window, some take off in a car, hard to say how it will play out.

Note to those who do consume or are around others who do: there is nothing you can do to stop this high, the person has to ride it out to the end. Inducing vomiting won't help and activated charcoal will do nothing. Your best response is to hydrate and try to keep the person calm and safe. If you are unable to maintain their immediate safety or if they are freaking out, get them to the hospital. Don't be surprised if there are several others in the waiting room experiencing the same thing.[3] The doctor will likely put the patient in bed, sometimes in restraints, and give them an antipsychotic medication while they hydrate and wait for the episode to calm down, in 12 hours or so.

One of the frustrating things about all of this is that we could easily cut THC overdoses way down if state lawmakers would firmly and knowledgeably stand up to the industry and implement some really simple rules, like one package, one dose. No longer could they sell a cake pop with 100 legal doses or a can of soda with 35 doses.

The other change needs to be a reexamination of the weight that is allowed per serving. If it is the dry weight of flowered cannabis baked into something, keep it at 10mg, whatever. But if it is a concentrate (and it's almost all concentrates) then it has to be adjusted down. To keep the math simple use 10% as the assumed potency of flowered cannabis. If an edible is infused with a 50% concentrate, lower the allowance to 5mg's, if 99.9% they 1mg per edible. The only reason I can imagine for not making these simple changes is caving under pressure from the THC lobby. How is it okay to put multiple servings inside of one piece of candy or one drink? It makes no rational sense.

Chronic consumers readily acknowledge this is an issue, according to sites like cannaconnection.com, hailmaryjane.com, sativauniversity.com, cannabis.info, wayofleaf.com, and leafy.com. The Guardian, on 11/19/18, published an unsettling story called "You're Not Going To Die: How to survive an edible overdose."[4] The gravity of this issue regarding potency and overdoses is becoming more obvious. While this book was being written, a story was circulating around the country about ten middle school kids in LA that were hospitalized after overdosing on edible, THC-infused products. Youtube and TikTok have many videos of kids eating edibles in school, so it isn't hard to guess how the kids in LA got the idea.

Thanks to an industry that capitalizes on overuse and abuse, more and more products make it mindlessly easy for people to use THC absolutely anywhere and not expect to be noticed. The rise of these items has hit vulnerable young people especially hard. A good friend and accomplished adolescent psychiatrist, Dr. Chris Thurstone, and I were giving a talk to parents of highschoolers. Dr. Thurstone said something that had a deep impact upon me. He was explaining the developing brain and how the frontal part of the human brain isn't developed until the mid 20's. That part of the brain allows for "executive thought." He described the young brain as having a giant gas pedal and no brake pedal. My explanation is a bit more crude than his, so see what you think. "The brain develops in three stages. The first stage makes sure you remember to breathe and run away from predators. Second stage tells you to keep the species going and feel good; eat, eat, eat / sex, sex, sex. The last stage is when you pause and consider what am I eating and who am I having sex with." The point is the same, we don't get our brake pedal or our thinking part until much later in life. This is why we have different laws for kids than adults. If given the option, the young brain will almost always assume risk and disregard consequences. This is one of the many reasons why we have to make it harder for kids to make decisions that will negatively impact them later in life, decisions like using THC while their brain is developing. Lawmakers need to consider this side of the coin when making rules for edibles, rather than simply garnering campaign contributions from the industry or accepting popular misconceptions about the risks. I believe regulating these products is essential to reduce and avoid overdose and youth use. To argue against more regulation is to parrot the industry talking points. Looking at the issues critically and thoughtfully are in everyone's best interests.

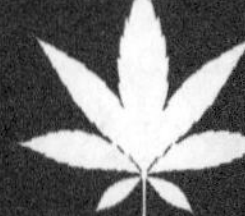

CHAPTER

08

MENTAL HEALTH

Mental Illness is to THC What Cancer Was to Tobacco, This Will be What Changes The Narrative

Recently, my wife asked if I was angry or disappointed by "nobody listening" to the public warnings we've been "shouting from the rooftops" regarding the issues that we are now dealing with around THC? The truth is that plenty of people have listened and the voices of those sounding the warning bells are growing daily. And, I believe, there is an awakening and a reckoning on the horizon.

There is a great untold story; a story that is as closely tied to weed as cancer is related to cigarettes. This untold story will ultimately dismantle the weed industry, but the issue is how much damage will we allow beforehand. Who ends up telling this untold story, social influencers, the pro-weed lobby, SAMHSA, the Surgeon General???

First, a bit of a history recap. My grandparents grew up believing cigarettes don't cause cancer. They believed this despite a warning issued in 1929 by the US Surgeon General, Hugh S. Cumming, describing the harms of smoking. It wasn't until a momentous report in 1964 from Surgeon General Luther Terry that America started to pay attention. At that time, people trusted the medical community a bit more and the report had a huge impact.

One of my closest friends has a dad named John. Their family included me in everything, even reunions, so I learned a lot of their stories. In 1964 John was rising through the ranks of the Air Force, where he would ultimately retire as a Lt. Colonel. John was a 2-plus pack a day smoker, waking up in the middle of the night for a smoke to stop the coughing and craving. The moment he read the 1964 report he put cigarettes down and never picked one up again. It was not only the risks to himself that made him stop, but it was reading about what it could do to his children that convinced him it simply wasn't worth it and he quit. Today the risks of smoking are universally understood and anyone who chooses to smoke does so with some knowledge of the risks detailed on the side of each cigarette pack. Simple brain development makes getting kids to start smoking early crucial to the future of the tobacco industry. Since people in the United States have pushed back on big tobacco, the companies have shifted their strategy to hooking people, especially young people, on their products in second and third world countries, where poverty has kept education years behind. The same thing will eventually happen with THC for another reason, **Mental Health**.

On 9/2/19, Surgeon General Admiral Vivek Murthy issued a report on the harms of THC. There were some real gems in the report including this: "While the perceived harm of marijuana is decreasing, the scary truth is that the actual potential for harm is increasing. And with marijuana now legalized to some degree in more than 30 states, consumers may underestimate the risks of this drug." The report also said, "This ain't your mother's marijuana. The higher the THC delivery, the higher the risk." This report has similarities to the statement from 1929 on tobacco.[1] With tobacco, it was another 35 years before the big report came out and moved the needle. How long will that period take with THC, will we need to wait for another report in 2054?

We are past the point of arguing about the connection between mental illness and THC. We are even past the point of wondering if it is just correlation or if causation exists. Right now, at the beginning of 2024, the untold story is this: <u>there is more than enough sound science to say that high potency THC is extremely damaging to the human brain and body.</u> The longer we wait the more the evidence will pile up. The issue is that in America it is believed that whoever has the loudest voice speaks the truth. Volume usually is dictated by money and there is no money to be made in prevention unless we play the long game and think about future consequences. A couple of things are going to happen: either the public health emergency becomes so large that it can no longer be ignored, OR huge sums of money will become available, like that which came after the class action suits and settlements against the tobacco companies. Increased capital will allow science to speak louder than sales and propaganda. We need accurate and compelling information coming from sources trusted enough today to accomplish what the Surgeon General did in 1964. Surprisingly, and I can't believe I'm saying this, the best hope we have for getting that kind of information to the public is through social media influencers! The unknown issue is whether influencers post things they believe in and care about or only things they are paid to promote. And, do influencers believe and care about things based upon evidence or only what they prefer to believe regardless of the facts? At some point the connection between mental illness and THC will be as widely known and accepted just as the connection between tobacco and cancer has become a reality. Science must win; my hope is that it does so quickly.

The first thing we have to do is establish a common and accurate understanding of the words we are about to consider. Let's begin with the word, "psychosis." The formal definition of this noun is "a severe mental disorder in which thought and emotions are so impaired that contact is lost with external reality." The professional world avoids pejorative terms, but in this case it seems appropriate to use the common term, "crazy." Crazy can look like lots of things, from paranoia to seeing and hearing things that nobody else fears, sees, or hears.

For illustration's sake, let's call psychosis "crazy town" and pretend that crazy town is a place on the map. There are two ways to get there: the organic or the chemical roads. Both end up in the same place. The organic route to crazy town is genetic; that was my path. With little to no mental illness on my dad's side and prolific mental illness on my mom's side, I was solidly predisposed to taking the organic route, it was in my genes.

The chemical route is when a person ends up in crazy town as a result of a substance(s). Until recently, much of drug induced psychosis was something that came about from amphetamines (meth and coke). Today it comes from THC. I want to be exceptionally clear about this, crazy town is not a good place to be in, so let's go back to calling it the right word, psychosis. Psychosis is not a good place to be. For those of you who have not seen psychosis there can be a tendency to downplay the awful reality of it. To the uninformed or the hard-hearted, a person in a psychotic state may seem amusing. Hopefully, those people stop laughing when they realize what is actually happening, that the person is detached from reality. If you are interested in seeing psychosis for real, search youtube. Please do so with this warning, these things can be very hard to watch and there is nothing at all funny about them.

Here is something else to consider, one can have a psychotic episode or a psychotic break. An episode has an ending, a break is when something shifts permanently in the brain and it will never be the same. The difference is whether the person is visiting crazy town or moving there. With this working understanding of psychosis we will examine it in more detail.

Cannabis or THC induced psychosis is not only on the rise, it is showing up so often that my friend Roneet Lev, an emergency room physician in California, expects to see cases of THC poisoning on every single shift she works. Dr. Lev gave me the following quote "The greatest problem our emergency departments have is boarding people in the emergency department. These are people who live in the ER for days, weeks and months waiting for a mental health bed. Many of these are detoxifying from cannabis."

A quick search of academia.edu turns up 24,635 scholarly articles with "cannabis" and "Psychosis" in the title. That number goes down to 23 citations when only considering papers from the last two years. Unfortunately, many searches do not include what many consider to be the landmark study on this issue, "Gone to Pot – A Review of the Association between Cannabis and Psychosis," originally published 5/22/14 by Rajiv Radhakrishnan, Samuel T. Wilkinson, and Deepak Cyril D'Souza. The citations alone take multiple pages to include the 358 JOURNAL PUBLISHED PEER REVIEWED studies that are mentioned within the paper. Assuming most will not read this paper in its entirety, here is a key portion of the conclusion:

'In the United States, the legal status of cannabis for medical and recreational purposes is changing rapidly. Pertinent findings that are likely to impact public health include high conversion rates from cannabis-induced psychosis to schizophrenia; global and specific domains of cognitive impairment resulting from cannabis use, which may be irreversible; the effects of acute intoxication; the precipitation of psychotic disorders in genetically vulnerable populations, including individuals with a history of childhood abuse or family history of psychotic disorders; and the increased risk of negative effects of cannabis use in prolonged and early exposure.[2]

Another very interesting study is one from 2012 entitled "Acute effects of a single, oral dose of d9-tetrahydrocannabinol (THC) and cannabidiol (CBD) administration in healthy volunteers" What makes this so important is the use of a true double blind placebo controlled study, the gold standard for solid science and something we need much more of. The other interesting thing to note is that they were using 10mg of THC as a "dose" but the potency is unspecified. To again save you from reading this in its entirety a quote from the Conclusion:

"(The) administration of THC was associated with anxiety, dysphoria, positive psychotic symptoms, physical and mental sedation, subjective intoxication

They go on to say that there were no issues associated with the CBD dose.[3]

One of the age old questions regards causation versus correlation; does THC cause psychosis or do more people with psychosis use THC? My friend Kevin Sabet says it best when explaining this question to those of us who aren't Fulbright Scholars, "More people eat ice cream in the summer, there are more murders in cities in the summer, does that mean that ice cream causes murders?" Of course not, this is an example of simple correlation. But every time my son is directly exposed to nuts he will have an anaphylactic reaction. He is allergic to nuts therefore the nuts are causal to his allergic reaction.

So back to the question at hand, does THC cause psychosis? The answer appears to be yes with continuing clarity as time goes on and more evidence is gathered. It is very important to note here that the majority of people who use THC will not experience psychosis. In a similar way, the majority of people who are lifetime smokers will not get lung cancer, but in the 10-20% who do get cancer it is also causal; it was tied to their genetics.[4] Thankfully today we have more than enough data and public understanding. Anyone who chooses to smoke is doing so with the risks well understood. The same universal understanding must be achieved among THC users.

The study most cited on the causation topic at this point is, "The contribution of cannabis use to variation in the incidence of psychotic disorder across Europe (EU-GEI): a multicentre case-control study." From the Lancet, May 1 2009, comes this about the '09 study:

> This 5 year study had an impressive N (number of subjects) of 1130. It also considered "high potency" THC 10-16%. There is so much that can be learned from this study but for our purposes the most interesting is that the risk of psychosis doubles when use is initiated by 15 years old if it is high potency being consumed and almost no change if THC is under 10%. This study shows us that THC potency under 10% is relatively harmless, relatively, while over 10% is causing and increasing psychosis. Simple math, keep it under 10% and things are cool for the user, unfortunately less cool for the supplier. Earlier in the study they say something very interesting: "Those who spent €20 or more a week showed more than a doubling in the odds of a psychotic disorder."[5] My case from earlier is again validated, the money is in the problem user and the industry cares not about the individual but about their wallet.

Another idea that I would like to consider here is suicide. Data lags so the best we have is 2021 and it is the highest ever recorded in Colorado history according to CDPHE. The same data records the highest rates of teen suicide we have ever seen.[6] While there is some science starting to point towards causation, I am not ready to make that claim. However, based on multiple studies including:

- Associations of Suicidality Trends With Cannabis Use as a Function of Sex and Depression Status (2021)[7]
- Young adult sequelae of adolescent cannabis use: an integrative analysis (2014)[8]

I am absolutely ready to point out the correlation between THC and suicide. Given the severity of what we are discussing, suicide, it is of utmost importance that we discourage use, especially youth use, until more is known.

There is much more solid data on this subject, but it is beyond the pale of this book. Go to www.iasic1.org (INTERNATIONAL ACADEMY ON THE SCIENCE AND IMPACT OF CANNABIS) and head to their "library." They have a huge database.

The bottomline is that the connection of THC and psychosis has been observed as early as the 1600's. Now, causality is established; high potency THC being much worse.[9] As someone who has struggled with mental illness personally and witnessed first hand much more than I can quantify, it makes me so sad that we are ignoring this issue, and to our peril. The undeniable scientific truth will win the day, but will we allow this to again mimic big tobacco in the amount of time it takes to react or will we take some action?

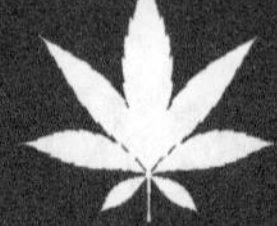

CHAPTER

09

'MERICA!

F Ya!

"What about Uruguay, or Amsterdam, things are good there!" I hear a variation of that as often as I ask my wife where my car keys are, and that's a lot. People are always trying to compare our country to those two. The following is meant to address these issues.

First, let's begin by saying America isn't like Uruguay or Amsterdam, like not at all. In America we supersize our big macs. In America we drive our kids to school in 700hp trucks that get 10mpg. In America we sell our beer in 40 oz bottles. In America we order dessert first and get fast food because "you deserve a break today." In America, our weed makes "their" weed look like nothing. We are a nation of more, bigger and faster. Prudence and self restraint are not really our things, neither is good regulation.

Uruguay is a nation of about 3.5 million people where 32% are professing Catholics and 8% are evangelicals.[1] It is the population of Connecticut with the religious makeup of New York-ish. Weed is totally legal there and has been since 2012. Before it was legalized, it had never been criminalized. There was no black market nor was there a big commercial interest driving the conversation. In Uruguay, you can grow a few plants and they even have "social clubs" where people can use marijuana in a group setting. The government controls the price in order to keep it from getting too high and empowering the black market although there has been no decrease in the black market. 7/10 is the amount of people in Uruguay who buy their weed on the black market.[2] When the market first opened, potency was capped at 9% THC, with a minimum of 3% CBD. Recently advocates for unnaturally potent weed have pushed that cap to 15% (like in Amsterdam). To purchase weed in Uruguay you must be a resident; visitors to the country may not purchase.

According to a report from May 2022 there are about 32,000 registered users in Uruguay (.009 of the population) and they are limited to 1.4oz/month.[3] While they still lack some fundamental testing and consumer protections, this country went about it carefully, building a process for sales controlled by the government and limiting the potency in order to reduce harm. This is a reasonable approach, versus our hyper-caffeinated teenager way of going about it in the US. Uruguay stands out as a mostly careful and thoughtful way to change drug policy, but our profiteers tell the story of how great it is there without mentioning the closely controlled regulations. It's a bit like telling the story of Jack and the Beanstalk without the giant! It was so awesome for Jack, he just climbed up this magic plant, scored a singing harp and a goose that laid golden eggs and came home to his loving mother! From that day forward he had all the beans he could eat, all the gold he could spend and a weird harp that creeped people out when they visited. But that's NOT the whole story! We accept only the good parts from a story and ignore the negative to our peril.

Amsterdam is another place people love to talk about. One of my favorite parts about their weed laws is that it is expressly illegal to advertise, including online. Another good thing is that in 2011 they identified cannabis above 15% potency as a "hard drug," rather than its former classification as a "soft drug."[4] Soft drugs have a very different set of rules than hard drugs, which include meth and cocaine. Amsterdam recently banned the consumption of weed in public, even in the redlight district![5] It's significant that in a place where you can walk the streets and pick out women to buy sex from in windows, the residents banned smoking THC in order to "improve quality of life."[6] Additionally, the Netherlands have aggressive interventions aimed at helping people who have crossed the line from use to addiction, something this country hasn't even seriously considered. Despite lots of talk about using all those tax dollars for treatment and prevention, we don't. The state of public funding for mental health, including addiction in the US (unlike the Netherlands) is a sad joke; ask anyone who has tried to get a loved one care.

The intent of this chapter is not to highlight other nations and their policies, Rather, the purpose in giving these two examples is to demonstrate how irrational and pitifully inadequate our policies, regulations, and interventions are. Our approach has been one of "ready, shoot, aim" when dealing with individual and public health. We tend to make reactionary laws because something happened to someone who got on TV, rather than follow the science and make policy based on the facts. Over the years we have given corporations rights above those of the citizens and in doing so, created a nation where the corporate interest enjoys the same protections as the rest of us but they have way more money to get the laws they want put into place.[7] The laws that they want are predictably favorable towards making more money and then influencing more laws. To profiteers, we are just a member of one demographic or another, and we are consumers, from whom they seek to get money by almost any means.

I will again make the point that there are no immediate, short-term financial benefits when preventing addiction and mental illness. However, the long term gains are easily measured and well understood. In a world where political leaders see the world in 2-4 year election cycles, and in a culture where time is money and immediate gratification is a fundamental right, there is little incentive to pursue prevention. The educated consumer is like David with a slingshot and the Weed industry is Goliath with all the powerful resources. However, preventing and providing addiction treatment can be profitable. It's time for full disclosure and disclaimer.

Providing addiction treatment is my business, and the more addiction there is the better our business. It is not in my best financial interests to oppose ineffective drug laws, like those in this country pertaining to THC commercialization, but I do oppose them in the strongest way. Yes, there are plenty of people in the recovery business who do it for the wrong reasons, but there are many, including myself, in our field who desire collective health and wellness over personal profit. The day I wake up and there is no need for me to do what I do anymore will be the best day of my life. But I say that, sadly, knowing that day will not come. I also want to be clear that I prefer our free market system to the failed attempts at socialized interventions, but I do think the market should have some checks and balances. The US currently enjoys the distinction of having the highest rates of drug use in the world. That's not a distinction anyone should want. And we are ranked 27th in the world for "healthcare and education."[8] Is it reasonable to think that if the first would decrease the second might increase?

By sanctioning another intoxicating and addictive substance, and worst of all by failing to regulate it, we see another unfortunate and dangerous demonstration of profit over people. If we continue along the current path our nation will continue its downward slide.

The other day I had some work to do in Florida, a talk for a community group. Since it had been a nasty winter at home with a couple of months left on it I decided to stay the weekend and go fishing in the sun. One of my best friends flew in and we headed down to Islamorada in the Keys to chase Tarpon. Throughout the trip our guide was pointing out boats, some offshore and some beached, that bring the 200-300 Cuban and Haitian migrants a day. These vessels were amazing to see, none seemed seaworthy enough to make the 80 mile voyage. One even appeared to be made of foam and tarps. A small sailboat several hundred yards from shore was unloading its human cargo. The guide estimated that the 30-some foot craft had 250 people on board. There were children everywhere and not a single lifejacket to be seen. I asked him what these people did if they made it. After explaining the legal processes involved, he said that 80% or more go straight to work and "work their asses off." Those who employ people are desperate to find hard-working people to employ. This nation is still so amazing and full of opportunity that hundreds of people are willing to risk their lives crossing the Atlantic from Cuba each day just for a chance to be a part of the United States. I hope they aren't disappointed when they realize that many would rather be drunk and stoned than demand some accountability from those who govern us. Don't get me wrong, I'm not one of those 'America was better back in the day' guys who whitewash the awful things that have taken place here, but I do believe that we used to contribute more and read more than get high.

The amazing trust that advocates for drugs seem to have in our government and corporate sector is striking. For instance, consider Doug Fine. He lives in New Mexico and writes books. In addition to being a "Best Selling Author," Doug describes himself as a "Solar Powered Goat-Herder" and goes to great lengths to validate his hippy/counter culture credentials. Doug is a perfect case study in this issue. He is someone who on the surface would reject big business and big government yet is advocating for both in his outspoken support for the weed industry. Here are a few quotes from a chapter entitled "Redneck Hippie Capitalism"(emphasis mine):

"...Big Money and Big Law were prepared to bankroll Mendocino's idea of sustainable cannabis..." It occurred to me that perhaps it was time for me to get over my own lingering sense of culture war stigma surrounding this plant. Not only is it actually vital medicine for many, not only is it a potential source, through industrial biofuel, for America's energy needs, **but it might be where I should be directing my broker since it is clearly viewed to be an extremely profitable 'investment space to a lot of high-end venture capital."**

In the "Afterword" of the book Doug writes,: "Colorado's new law, vitally also allows industrial cannabis cultivation" and "Cannabis is to American agriculture today is what Silicon Valley was to American Industry in the 1970's"[9]

The main takeaway from his writing is the belief that there's just too much money to be made in weed for us not to bring it into the mainstream and give it to big business and put it under control of the government. I disagree with this premise for a number of reasons. First, we must be concerned with more than just finances and the bottom line. Because something is profitable doesn't make it right or just; look at slavery, opiate mills, war.

The other point has been mentioned before; are state and or federal government(s) capable and willing to appropriately regulate THC? Past examples of regulation around alcohol, tobacco, firearms, healthcare, etc. would be laughable were they not so serious and harmful. The task of appropriately regulating and doing quality control around THC will be a BIG job, costing lots of money, and taking strong leadership. Yet I continue to hear people, who I would have expected to have little trust in the government, encourage government regulation. This apparent contradiction gets unraveled with one or a combo of explanations:

1. It's a simple talking point that nobody has thought through, beyond the "tax and regulate" signs they carry.

2. People don't actually want safe, regulated THC, they just want to get high.

3. (My money is on this one.) The weed industry knows how impotent our government is and how easy it is to buy both time and laws. They have been counting on Uncle Sam turning a blind eye, so long as the outstretched hand doesn't go empty.

To underscore a point, we have no demonstrated history of designating massive resources to the regulation of products similar to THC.

In my last book I found out pre-publication that I had contractually obligated myself to providing them with an image of me for marketing. I am private and thought myself witty when i gave them a picture that my then 12-year old son drew of me. One of the things that people often assume when they meet me or see an image or video is that I kind of look like a clean cut pro business government supporting citizen, this can be credited to my rule that all tattoos must be concealable with business attire. People I discuss/argue this subject with often present as very counter-culture yet we find ourselves with me arguing against business and government oversight and them for it. This may seem to be in conflict from the earlier recommendations for federal oversight of marketing THC. Please remember, I don't think selling THC is a good idea at all, but if we are actually serious about doing this it has to be the responsibility of the federal government to regulate and enforce.

Supporting "legalization" in its current form is to support Big Business, Wall Street, Multinational firms, venture capitalists and political carpetbaggers. Decriminalizing accomplishes everything proponents say they want without the rich getting richer and the government embarrassing itself. But in America, we do what we want to do and, more often than not, what we 'want' is what the corporate powers tell us to want.

CHAPTER 10

ENVIRONMENT

Why We Should All Care

S ome questions to consider and issues to be grappled with:

Why are we not talking about the environmental impact of growing so much cannabis? When people in the American West can't water their lawns, why isn't anyone looking at and talking about how much the weed corporations are sucking up from the water supply?

Why are more outdoors people not up in arms about the damage being done to our public lands and waterways from the black-market growing sites that are flourishing under commercialization?

How is it that in California they have to warn you that parts of your car may cause cancer, but nobody is concerned about all of the chemicals and heavy metals being smoked and vaporized in commercially sold THC products?

How is it that we are so concerned with our individual energy consumption and in lowering our carbon footprint, but the energy-hungry indoor growing operations take up a huge portion of our grid?

These are big, unaddressed issues regarding THC and the environment. They are interrelated but will be handled individually. Let's begin with water consumption.

Opinions vary but the folks at "Royal Queen Seeds" seem to have put some real thought into their recommendations regarding water consumption and growing. They say that for every processed 500g of flower it takes 4.5 liters of water a day.[1]

According to some irrigation specialists, who did all kinds of math to make their determination, a cannabis plant needs .36 inches of water/day.[2]

The folks at MJBiz Daily cite a report from the "Journal of Cannabis Research." It claims that for every 100 sq/ft of indoor growing space, 22 gallons of water is needed a day and 22.1 gallons for the same space outdoors. This article goes on to get a bit more specific in saying that 22.7 liters or about 6 gallons of water is needed per day in an average growing season of 150 days.[3,4]

These measurements are nice because we're looking at three different ways to consider water usage, per processed weight, per inch and while growing. Let's put that into perspective by considering the amount of growing taking place.

According to the MED, Colorado produced 1.24 million plants, which equates to 662.3 metric tons of weed in 2020, it would appear that there are about 1,245 registered grows in Colorado, the largest of which is "Mammoth Farms" which maintains 3,484,800 sq/ft of growing.[5,6,7] Finding many more specifics about the size of grows in Colorado proves elusive. After finding a list of all licensed grow operations, I was unable to determine the size of those grows. I did find a list of the 20 largest grows in North America.[8] Once the seven Canadian growers were eliminated from the list, something interesting jumped out. The 13 largest grows in the country are all in the West, with the exception of Illinois. The remaining 12 are all in CA, CO, NM, AZ, and NV; all states listed as being in some form of drought.[9] That means the 13 largest grows with one exception are all located in drought areas and are collectively watering 46,865,739 sq/ft of weed. So here is our math story problem: If the 13 largest cannabis grows in the US total 46,865,739 sq/ft and it takes 22 gallons of water a day to water 100 sq/ft how much water is being used per day to support those private companies? *Don't forget to show your work!*

46,865,739 sq. ft. / 100 sq. ft. = 468,657.39 sq. ft.

468,657.39 sq. ft. x 22 gal. = 10,310,426 gallons

Answer: The thirteen largest grow operations in the US consume 10,310,426 gallons of water a day!

The average American household consumes 300 gallons of water a day.[10] Which means that the 13 largest grows in the country use as much water as 34,368 average households.

Let's work on another math problem using total grown cannabis in the US. According to a report by Whitney Economics, the US grew 48.8 million pounds in 2022.[11-]

If the US produces 48,800,000 lbs of cannabis in 2023 and there are 453.592 grams in a pound. Each 500 grams uses 4.6 liters of water and there are 3.78541 liters to a gallon, then how many gallons of water will America use to get high on THC in 2023?

Don't forget to show your work!

48,800,000 lbs. x 453.592 gr. = 22,135,289,600 grams
22,135,289,600 gr. / 500 gr. = 44,270,579.2 grams
44,270,579.2 gr. x 4.6 ltrs. = 203,644,664 liters
203,644,664 ltrs. / 3.78541 lits. = 53,797,228.8 gallons
53,797,228.8 gal. x 365 days = 19,635,988,512 gallons in 2023

Bonus question: If the average US home uses 300 gallons of water a day how many homes could be supplied per day with the water it takes to grow weed?

53,797,228.8 / 300 = 179,324 homes

Growing all of this weed is devastating our water supply and mostly in places that don't have the water to spare. It is outside the scope of this book to get into the issues with all of the black market grows. Let it be said that they have increased tremendously since commercialization, and the destruction they are causing is significant. This must be addressed.[12]

One last thing about water before I go onto the next environmental issue with this industry. Water coming out the back end of the growing process is seriously tainted. The influence of pesticides and fertilizers will be highlighted later. For now it is sufficient to know that the water draining from these GMO plants is not usable, by anyone for anything. By the time growers are done pumping steroids into their cloned marijuana plants, much of that garbage has saturated the wastewater, which would require serious efforts to clean it up.

The water we use for outdoor crops, watering our lawns, etc. is absorbed back into the ground or evaporates to be recycled as rain/humidity/dew. While it's important to be very careful with this resource, especially in dry places, most of the water used for irrigation returns to the water table in pretty short order. That's not the case with weed water! Weed water is a corrupted sludge-like substance that takes a very long time to return to a state where it can reenter the water table.

So to summarize these issues, marijuana production not only uses water we don't really have, it also allows multistate and multinational companies doing the growing to destroy water supplies without doing anything to help prevent or treat it. I kind of like that visual now that I write it! Picture us (America) all drinking out of a kiddie swimming pool and while most are using spoons to sip, the THC companies are scooping their water up in cups and simultaneously peeing it back into the pool. If you need a little more detail to make the image complete the guy you are picturing as the THC industry should be in awful physical shape but wearing a very nice suit and watch.

The next big environmental concern is power. Back in the olden days, when weed grew outside and naturally, all the power that was needed was the sun. It was free and sunlight is infinitely renewable. Between the time that it rises in the east and sets in the west, the sun provides power in many forms, including photosynthesis and plant growth.

For quite a while, people have been growing weed indoors. The key advantage was making it harder to get caught. Before the laws changed and made it legal to grow outdoors, law enforcement was able to catch people illegally growing weed indoors by keeping an eye on the grid and knocking on doors of places that were using WAY more power than they should be using. Growing inside requires grow lamps in place of sunlight and they consume a lot of power. In addition to the lamps, there is the huge power usage coming from the air exchange that has to take place inside indoor growing operations. With all of those lights it gets super hot and that heat has to be evacuated, which means state of the art, and very power hungry, air circulation systems.

In my last book, Evan Mills, PhD did the math and provided a great paper showing that about 1% of the US grid would go to growing commercial weed in 2011.[14] Running the numbers again in 2023 is startling. Colorado State University researchers released a paper in the Journal of Nature and Sustainability in July of 2021 that gave us a comprehensive equation of energy used to produce weed. Their formula considers all regions of the country and averages power use to give us 3,658 kgCO2e kg.[15] Using that figure as well as the number we used above to calculate water usage of projected total corporate growth as well as what the EPA tells us cars use, the weed grown in 2023 is equal to burning 196,716,479,138,872 gallons of gas through an average US vehicle. I wasn't sure what a number with 15 digits was even called, turns out it is hundred trillions, thanks Google. If you want to say this in a sentence here it is: Commercially grown weed in the United States will use the same Co2 as one hundred ninety-six trillion, seven hundred sixteen billion, four hundred seventy-nine million, one hundred thirty-eight thousand, eight hundred seventy-two gallons of gas driven in the average vehicle. Or 196.7 trillion gallons. Lake Erie holds 127.6 trillion gallons.

Now, let's apply "apples to apples." Although Dr. Mills has not updated his paper, he continues to write a great deal on the subject. (I salute his free thinking approach and his willingness to question the system.) Using the projected number of 2023 growing, 48.8 million, and applying the average number of 2,500, which is the commonly accepted 2-3k kilowatt hours it takes to grow one pound of weed, as well as the projected usage of energy in the US this year of 4,172,000,000,000 KWh, it would appear that about 2.9% of the US grid will go towards growing weed, about triple what it was when I last wrote![16]

The THC lobby will want to argue that the power was being used before but secretly; now it's above board with good law abiding drug traffickers. The big issue with this argument is that not only has the black market not disappeared as promised, it has grown under commercialization, so both legal and illegal operations are consuming large amounts of the electrical grid. We have not exposed the use of these finite resources by the weed industry, we have added to them.

There are constant reminders that we are running out of clean, renewable water in much of this country. The weed industry increases and accelerates that problem, all for the sake of getting high! This industry is one more example of big business using WAY more than their fair share of water and power, as well as polluting, and then making a huge deal when their newest "Green initiative" makes them appear virtuous.

In America, we get to do what we want, for the most part. But it's important that we know what we're demanding of the planet, especially if you chose to buy THC. Remember the immortal words of Captain Planet "The power is yours."

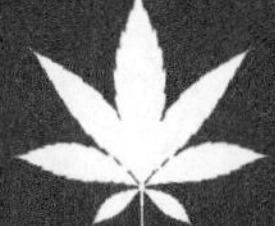

CHAPTER

11

MEDICINE AND SCIENCE AND SHIT

There Is Much More Known Than We Are Led To Believe

"Do you support medical marijuana?," I am often asked. "Of course I do, I'm a big fan of medicine," but it's critical that we know what "medical marijuana" actually is. The difference between medical marijuana and recreational marijuana, and this may surprise you, is taxes. In most states in the US where one can purchase both medical and recreational marijuana, the products are exactly the same. But you pay less in taxes if you have a med card. Otherwise, the products are exactly the same. Going back to the first chapter where we talked about the importance of language, something to be called "medicine" should be approved as such.

As I write this there are four medications that are cannabis based:

Cesamet (nabilone, a synthetic cannabinoid similar to THC) – Available in the U.S.[1]

Epidiolex (a plant-derived CBD) – Available in the U.S.[2]

Marinol (dronabinol, a synthetic THC) – Available in the U.S.[3]

Sativex (a combination of THC and CBD in a 1:1 ratio) is a prescription cannabinoid available in Canada and Europe but not yet FDA-approved or available in the U.S.[4]

Although Sativex is not yet found in the US, it has some compelling studies behind it as do the others. Epidiolex is the medicine that I hear talked about most often and I encourage people to talk to their doctors about Epidiolex for more information. It seems that many people are excited about CBD nowadays and always want to talk about it. There is a big problem with CBD that I will elaborate on soon, which makes Epidiolex the only reliable form of CBD available. Epidiolex is only FDA approved for some rare seizure disorders, but it can be prescribed off label, which some doctors are willing to do. There are a few potential side effects with this medication, as with all, but we know these include: loss of appetite, nausea, vomiting, fever, feeling unwell, unusual tiredness, yellowing of the skin or the whites of the eyes (jaundice), itching, unusual darkening of the urine, right upper stomach area pain or discomfort.[5]

This medication, along with all other medicines, lists potential side effects. When it comes to "medical" marijuana, producers and dispensaries simply don't do it. As mentioned before, this is a direct result of no oversight of the CBD industry. The issues that result from this lack of oversight are innumerable, here are a few.

Beginning with the example above, there is no requirement to report on side effects, therefore the industry doesn't. Refer to the list under "Mental Health" and you see why. People taking medicine have a right to understand the risks that are associated with that medication.

The other thing about Epidiolex we can tell you for sure is that most people start with a dose of 2.5mg/twice daily and scale up to 10-12mg. When it comes to other products, how much CBD is a "dose"? Most sellers will tell you to take a bunch of whatever it is because then you will be back sooner for more. But there are some issues with over consumption that we are starting to find out about. For instance, a study in mice suggests higher doses of CBD can do damage to livers.[6] One again, it's important, when taking a medication, to know how much to take. Many medications can become lethal in amounts too high.

Now for the drug/drug interactions. Doctors always check on other medications you are taking before putting you on something new. This is because many drugs interact with other drugs, some in acceptable ways, some in negative ways. CBD, for example, has known interactions with 585 other drugs, some of which can be serious. In fact, 15 of these drug interactions are considered "major" and 517 are labeled as "moderate." The definition of "major" is, "Highly clinically significant. Avoid combinations; the risk of the interaction outweighs the benefit." And "moderate" is defined as, "Moderately clinically significant. Usually avoid combinations; use it only under special circumstances."[7] These warnings are serious and consumers should be encouraged to pay attention to them.

Next on the list of problems has to do with people selling whatever they want and calling it CBD. There is literally nobody overseeing this gigantic industry, nobody. A study in 2017 showed that less than 31% of the tested CBD products were accurately labeled.[8] The problem is actually a good deal larger than that. Mislabeling is bad but selling dangerous products is worse. In order to make things clear, let's introduce this chapter's new vocabulary word," bioaccumulator." Webster defines this 7-syllable word as "the accumulation over time of a substance and especially a contaminant (such as a pesticide or heavy metal) in a living organism." Basically, a bioaccumulator is highly effective at absorbing and retaining contaminants, like heavy metals and pesticides. In 2022 an article highlighted some of the dangerous things found in CBD products being sold in stores, many of them edible. Out of a sample of 121 edible CBD products, lead was detected in 42%, cadmium in 8%, arsenic in 28%, and 37% contained mercury. Of the 516 products tested in the same study for accuracy, 40% contained less than 90% of the CBD indicated on the product label, 18% contained more than 110% of the labeled amount, and only 42% of products fell within plus/minus 10% of the CBD claimed on the manufacturer's label.[9]

Another study from 2020 revealed that of the 25 commercially purchased products tested, only three were within plus/minus 20% of the claim on their label. Fifteen were well below the stated claim for CBD; two exceeded claims in excess of 50%; and 5 made no claims. In addition, THC content for three products exceeded the 0.3% legal limit.[10] There are multiple studies and examples of this blatant mislabeling. The point is well-documented: without oversight there can be no reliable labeling, the industry has zero incentive to do so.

In that same vein, there are too many vague and often nonsensical words used to describe products with some kind of cannabis related ingredient in them. Let's look at some of the more outstanding examples. There is "cbd infused" clothing. This is not about the hemp t-shirts or hemp-made shoes that are available. Rather, there are companies saying that infusing their clothing with CBD will reduce fatigue and soreness when worn. Acabada is charging a premium ($125 for a sports bra to $180 for leggings and $240 for a jacket) for what they call CBD infused clothing.[11] There is another company called NUFABRX that sells CBD infused gear including a "neck towel" for $25.[12] There are more examples of this kind of misuse, abuse, dishonesty. "A fool and their money are easily separated," as the old saying goes. My favorite part about these products is how totally impossible it is to verify the claims of the manufacturers. It is simple market exploitation, and without oversight, people can be easily duped.

There is another great marketing phrase, "Hemp Infused." This too can mean ANYTHING. Someone could claim a lotion to be hemp infused by dropping half a hemp leaf in a big vat of lotion! Add the picture of the popular weed leaf on the package and you can add 50% to the price tag. Don't forget to make sure that what you are buying is "full-Spectrum." This means it contains everything found within the plant, including pesticides, fertilizers and heavy metals. Drop a trace amount of a hemp or cannabis plant into whatever it is you're making and it becomes "full-Spectrum."

The point is that CBD infused, Hemp infused, etc. means nothing. For those who protest saying, "This CBD cream is the only thing that has ever worked," there is the powerful effect of the placebo suggestion. An article in Medical News Today quotes oncologist Robert Bucknam as saying, "Placebos are extraordinary drugs. They seem to have some effect on almost every symptom known to mankind, and work in at least a third of patients and sometimes in up to 60 percent."[13]

If someone claims their CBD is making them feel better, that's fine. All I ask is that they talk about it with their doctor in case they are taking something that could potentially cause them harm.

Now for the nefarious effects of this unregulated industry. There are plenty of people taking what they believe to be CBD in place of the things their doctors want them to take. Many of these people are very sick and their conditions can be made worse by ingesting these mislabeled or unlabeled products.. There are lots of examples but the one closest to my heart is when people with PTSD are told to take something that very well may make their conditions worse. I doubt actual CBD would do much harm, and might even help if they think it will help, but what if it has THC in it? We know THC negatively affects PTSD.[14] Unscrupulous people try to sell more THC and CBD hiding behind very sick people, claiming their latest batch of unregulated whatever is the silver bullet. Some of those sufferers may actually benefit from medical grade CBD, like Epidiolex, but these marketers aren't interested in giving people medicine, they want them to buy their products. Profiteers, under the guise of advocates, will insist that the only way to treat many illnesses is with an unproven, unregulated and mostly mislabeled product, that they just so happen to sell. Modern day "snake oil."

One last point before moving on; CBD is what is called "hydrophobic." This means that it doesn't bind to or dissolve in liquid. While it can be forced to bind using nanotechnology, please ask yourself how many of the CBD drinks you are seeing in the gas station for $1 are using nanotechnology when they don't have to.

I was giving a talk not too long ago to a highschool when a student tried to make a mic drop moment. She asked me why, if THC was so damaging, were so many doctors prescribing it to kids with mental health disorders like depression, anxiety, PTSD, etc. When the shouting and chest bumping subsided I answered, first by complementing the young lady for having the guts to stand up and question an "expert" and told the kids how important I believe civil discourse to be. With that done I went on to explain that no doctor in the US ever "prescribed" cannabis to anyone, especially not a kid. Ya see, the trick is in the language, and we need to be much more careful with the language to avoid misconceptions like this young lady had. THC is a schedule 1 controlled substance. Schedule 1 drugs can not be prescribed, like ever. That is due to the definition of schedule 1 "drugs with no currently accepted medical use and a high potential for abuse."[15] Let me be very clear, I am not defending the classification of cannabis as a schedule 1 narcotic, but it is one, at least right now. Things that are not schedule 1 are cannabis derived drugs/medications, the reason being that they can be recreated with predictability whereas growing a plant can't. I would love for and have been advocating to have the components of cannabis be actually studied. Interestingly one of the biggest roadblocks to this has been the sellers of "medical marijuana"

The realm of medical marijuana and CBD presents challenges due to the lack of oversight, mislabeling, and potential risks associated with unregulated products. It is imperative that consumers, healthcare providers, and policymakers prioritize accurate information, responsible regulation, and scientific study. By doing so, we can promote the safe and effective use of cannabis-based medications while avoiding the exploitation of vulnerable populations.

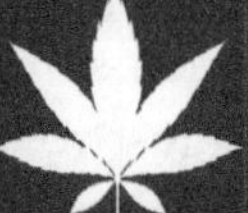

CHAPTER

12

ALL THE NONSENSE OR "THANK YOU 2018 FARM BILL"

Washington Is At It Again!

This chapter almost didn't get written, but it may help us know exactly what it is we are buying inside the local gas station for $3.99. Before looking into the chemistry we need to know, we have to go back a few years to when this all started, in 2018. Situations were such that it got pretty crucial that the Farm Bill get passed so it did, pork and all. There was some language in the Farm Bill that, when signed into law, opened a whole new Pandora's Box. What they did, either unintentionally (ignorance) or intentionally (devious) was to define "hemp" as anything measuring .3% THC or less.[1] In other words, they established a definition describing what weed wasn't. That left everything else to be qualified as "hemp" and therefore legal under the Farm Bill. Ignoring the key issue of enforcing regulations, let's focus on the actual changes that the law allowed.

Cannabis contains a lot of chemicals inside it, but the farm bill only specified one, "delta 9 THC." Some of the chemicals it didn't address, and therefore made legal to sell, were:

1. THC-A
2. THC-O
3. THC-P
4. THC-V
5. HHC
6. Delta 8
7. Delta 10

These chemicals can be delivered to any address in the country and purchased in smoke shops and gas stations in all 50 states.

THC-A

Basically THC-A doesn't produce a "high" because it can't bind to the receptors in the brain that produce that response.. It's found in cannabis as the acidic form of THC. No one would care about THC-A since it cannot produce a high. But with the help of basic science, THC-A can be converted into Delta 9 THC (the stuff that gets you high). At about 200 degrees, all you have to do is smoke or vape THC-A and what you bought as a non-intoxicating component of the plant becomes good old fashioned, high-producing Delta 9.[2]

THC-O

The reason why you are hearing more about this is because it is refuted to be about 3x as strong as regular, old THC. There are ample warnings about the strength of this chemical, but those warnings turn out to make for better advertisements than deterrents. To get THC-O one first must extract the Delta 8 and then run in through an intense, and HIGHLY flammable, chemical called Acetic Anhydride.[3] PubChem describes the chemical as being 'corrosive to metals and tissue' and can be used to make a few things including 'plastics and explosives.[4] Several retailers have recently stopped selling THC-O because of how dangerous it is to make and consume. Apparently heating THC-O causes the formation of Ketene which kills people when smoked or vaped. The descriptions online all compare its consistency to that of motor oil.

THC-P

This chemical is reserved for the big deal issues, or according to leafwell.com, for people who have substantial pain or cancer. Although it was just discovered in 2019 and with absolutely zero evidence, marketers are already suggesting it could be good to treat cancer. THC-P binds to your CB1 receptors much better than THC, 33x better. This has led to the common belief that it is 33x stronger than THC, so people with high tolerances love it.[5] Since it occurs in such small amounts naturally what you buy in the stores is going to be a lab synthesized chemical with the same makeup as what the plant has. So much for the "it's natural" argument.

THC-V

I doubt you will see much of this one because it does not appear to make you high and is very difficult to extract. The proposed upside to it is that people report it suppresses their appetites, so it is finding popularity in some circles.[6]

HHC

Adding hydrogen molecules to CBD produces HHC. The other ways it's being extracted today are proprietary, so people are tight lipped on it. Kyle Ray, chief operating officer of Colorado Chromatography, said the process takes place within a chemical reactor; "In goes CBD, out comes HHC." What's most interesting about HHC is that it's believed not to show up in a drug test. People like that part. It is also billed as "weed lite," something that gets you less intoxicated than THC.[7,8]

Delta-8

This is the one everyone is talking about, it's very much in fashion. Delta-8 is so well known that the FDA has even weighed in on it. Although they haven't taken the time to regulate it or anything silly like that, they did post this warning on their site. They go on to say "It is important for consumers to be aware that delta-8 THC products have not been evaluated or approved by the FDA for safe use in any context. They may be marketed in ways that put the public health at risk and should especially be kept out of reach of children and pets."[9]

The general consensus is that Delta-8 is like lite beer, it gets you high but not super high. It has to be produced in labs by pushing solvents through organic material.

Delta-10

This is pretty much the same as Delta-8, the main difference being that it isn't called, "Delta-8." It's made the same way and does the same thing, but as some states have started to crack down on, or at least pass laws restricting, Delta-8, Delta-10 has the distinct advantage of not being illegal under those laws.

As my good friend Duke likes to say, "Where are all the angry moms with pitchforks and torches!" In other words, where are the protests and pushback by parents and other concerned people regarding the impact of these chemicals on mental health and safety? Perhaps we think it's someone else's problem, the neighbor's kid is the one buying this stuff when they fill up at the local gas station. Unfortunately, many kids, perhaps our own, are buying these things. Why? Because they can. Federal inaction and poor policies, like the Farm Bill, have made this a reality.

CHAPTER 13

KIDS/PARENTS

For Those of You in the Struggle

A reporter from the New York Post recently called asking my thoughts on a bill that would require parents to attend diversion/education programs with their kids when the kids got caught with THC. While I like the idea of putting them all in the same room, my initial concern was what will the curriculum contain? How will the state create a class that will have information relevant to both parents and their kids? The challenge that this call brought to the forefront of my mind is how to bridge the gap between the perception of what kids are using and the reality of what is actually happening on the street. As I have suggested prior, we must start with a recognition that most parents will think of a plant while most kids will think of a product. My intention in this chapter is to better equip parents to have these conversations with their children in a way that will be meaningful. It is not enough to say something, we must say something that is true in a way that can be understood. I can do my best trying to discuss a subject in my native language, English, with someone who is a native speaker of say Mandarin, but no matter how hard I try and how earnest I am my message won't get through. For my words to mean anything they have to be understandable, factual and relevant.

I believe that the first thing we need to establish in these conversations is the difference between the plant and the products. By starting here we will be able to keep the conversation focused on the issue at hand and not the historical and societal problems associated with use and more importantly enforcement of laws. It is so easy for someone to gaslight in these conversations and change the conversation from one about themselves to one about Nixon era laws, or pervasive racism in American culture. The assumption I am making with this suggestion is that you are talking to someone for whom THC has become a problem. IF this is the case our primary practical concern is with their well being so we have to keep the conversation focused on their use.

This conversation is best conducted with three phases, the first of which is information gathering/understanding. By beginning your conversation this way you will avoid making it an accusation met by a rebuttal. Hopefully you will show the person that you care enough to learn about them before trying to "fix" them. The goal of this part of the conversation is to determine what is being used and how often. By "what" I mean potency and method of ingestion. Potency is key because it will allow us to get a better understanding of how severe the issue is or is not. If I find out that the person I'm talking to smokes joints rolled from dried out cannabis plants, I am less concerned than if they are vaping concentrates. The method of ingestion is also key to establish in part, so you don't sound stupid. You wouldn't want to be saying "smoking" when they are vaping or eating just like you wouldn't want to refer to the products as gummies when they smoke or vape. The way to ask this question is simple, "If you had a $1k gift card to your favorite dispensary, what would you walk out of the store with?" Get ready for some generic answers here, so probe a bit. If you hear things like "I don't know, some bud" or "a few cartridges" or "gummies and sodas," you will have to ask questions until you find out how strong those products are. If they say "bud" or "flower," ask specifically what strain. Ask if they prefer indica or sativa but most importantly find out how strong. A response might be something like, "Okay, so you prefer flower, what would the ideal THC amount be in that flower?" The same idea applies for vaping or edibles. Once you have a better idea of potency we want to shift to frequency. This one can be a bit trickier because pretty much everyone will downplay their use; you can typically multiply these answers by 2 and get closer to reality! The style and tone of the conversation will be a big factor in how honest an answer you are able to get.

Before moving on to phase two, let's be perfectly clear, ANY amount of use in the adolescent brain is problematic. Our concern for them increases the greater the potency is from zero and the frequency from never. As a general rule, potency above 10% and frequency over three times a month is when things become concerning. For example, if we find that someone is using a concentrate level potency (40%+ THC) multiple times a day our level of concern will be high. If they are smoking ditch weed once a month, I am far less concerned.

Phase two, compassionate concern. Keep in mind that you are having this conversation because you care about and love the individual and you want what is best for them. As a parent myself I understand how easy it is to confuse what I think is best for them with what they think is best. I encourage you to remember what it would have been like, or what it was like, having this conversation with your parents. Would you have been likely to respond well to, "You are an embarrassment and are throwing your life away. The Baker's kids would never do anything like this and they're all going places!" Or would your response be better to, "I hope you know how much I love you and that I always want the best for you no matter what life you lead. I am concerned that your use may be getting in the way of the future you want and of you being the person you want to be and doing the things you want to do."

There is a place for tough love and firm boundaries, but that place usually isn't in the first conversation about someone's use. Your goal here is to let them know you are concerned and that your concern comes from a place of love and caring, not from frustration and disappointment. Doing your best to keep anger in check will go a long way towards future conversations and ultimately the outcome.

Phase three is when we either suggest solutions or start looking for them. We'll call this the "solutions stage." Much of what comes next will depend on what has come up to this point. A flowchart to follow is not helpful because each situation is unique. Rather than establish specific interventions for each level of use I will suggest several responses, escalating from the least to the most serious.

- Agree to have another conversation

- Agree on boundaries specific to your situation and level of comfort; things like there is no use or possession in the home. Or they will stop using concentrates or not use more than once or twice a month.

- Agree to stop all use and to discuss it openly. One of the keys here is to agree to testing. The last thing you want is them being persecuted for something they didn't do or for you to figure out how to navigate the issues while being lied to.

- Talk to a professional. Getting a therapist or medical provider involved is only as good as that individual is in this field. I strongly suggest that you vet them first to make sure they are qualified and understand the issue. Unfortunately you will still find providers out there with the "It's just weed" mentality.

- Intensive OutPatient (IOP) therapy. This typically means three sessions a week about three hours in length complimented by at least a monthly individual session.

- Residential (inpatient) Center. These programs are for people who can't stop on their own and are having serious issues associated with their use.

- Acute Emergency Care. This almost always begins in the ER because the person is in immediate risk, psychologically or physically. Things like psychosis or serious GI issues like uncontrolled vomiting are reasons to seek emergency care. There are too many stories of people hurting themselves and others in a state of psychosis. If they are unsafe to get to an emergency room, call 911. If you call 911 make sure to explain that it is a psychiatric emergency and request a crisis response team. Many police departments now employ clinicians who will go on these calls to help de-escalate situations.

One final thought on having this conversation; don't do it in a time of crisis. If you initiate this when they come home past curfew, or you find a THC product in their room or right after another parent calls you with scary information, the conversation will miss its intended mark. These conversations are most impactful when things are "good," when everyone is well rested, fed, and emotions aren't flaring.

Okay parents, the easy part is done, let's talk about you! All those who parent run the risk of either catastrophizing or downplaying the situation. Either reaction can be a big problem. Consider if you will my contextual bias when it comes to these matters. I am a recovering addict who lost a majority of my youth's peer group to addiction. I also work inside of elective drug treatment where everyone has a severe addiction and is often near death. In my personal and professional experience, drug use leads to, as they say in 12-step, "jails institutions and death.'" In other words, the most serious of consequences. The challenge for me is to remember that my experience is not the whole sum of humanity's experience. There are plenty of people who will never experience what I did or see what I do at work; I have to keep that in mind. In the same way it is equally as important for those who use(d) or have people close to them who use to remember that what I see is also reality for some. Both of us have to avoid generalizing in order to fit our expectations.

As a parent or someone concerned for a loved one you are going to have to walk a difficult path between overreacting and downplaying; both can end in tragedy. Here are a few suggestions to help find this balance.

- Don't go it alone. We all have differing levels of support in our lives. Ideally you have a partner you can do this with, but for many that isn't a reality. Sometimes it is the partner that is the cause for concern. Reach out to friends and family, people you know are there for you. Talk to someone you know in recovery and ask them for advice or to people who have been in a similar situation as yourself. Talk to a therapist or leader in your faith community, if you have one. Attend a virtual or in person Al-Anon or Mar-Anon meeting and ask for help. (Mar-Anon is a support group for those who are affected by a loved one's marijuana use.)

- Don't be afraid to call in a professional prior to the conversation.

- Do your very best to be in a good place emotionally when you talk. Practice sound self care before walking into this.

- Stay pragmatic! You won't fix everything at once. Know the goal of the conversation (admit they need help, check into a program, agree to boundaries, etc) and stay focused on that. Far too often we want to have everything figured out. The goal is to get from point A to point B; we worry about C after that.

I will close this out by saying again that each and every situation is unique although they typically share some common themes. The only absolute thing to keep in mind is that someone is never too far gone to be helped. After working with families in the most desperate of situations, I always encourage them to not lose hope. This doesn't mean that you keep supporting and enabling a person, what it means is that you don't give up on them.

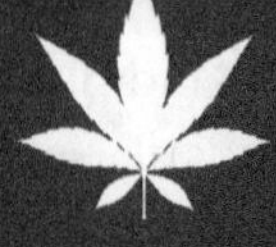

CHAPTER

14

TO THE PROVIDER

What We Need To Know To Treat

When I wrote the last book it was an effort to stop traveling and speaking so often. It turned out to accomplish the opposite. I have a job that keeps me busy so I try to avoid traveling to speak when I can but one thing that will get me on a plane quickly is when someone has a CEU/CME event for clinicians or medical providers. The gap in knowledge that many providers have on this subject often can lead to inadequate care, or no care at all. We need to be better educated and prepared to deal with the Cannabis Use Disorder (CUD) and Cannabis Withdraw Syndrome (CWS) that is showing up more and more frequently.

Before diving into this subject, let me warn the reader that what follows is primarily intended for front line providers, so if you are not in that role this part might not mean much to you. I'm going to use language familiar to us in the field and focus on treatment, so feel free to skip this chapter if it isn't for you.

Let me begin by suggesting that you purchase a book: <u>Cannabis in Medicine an Evidence Based Approach</u>, edited by Ken Finn MD and with lots of contributors, from Springer Publishing, 2020.[1] Dr Finn was asked to compile this textbook with consideration to multiple subspecialties of medicine. Ken called me several years ago and asked if I would write the chapter on treatment and recovery. I was honored for a second then intimidated, I would be the only non MD/DO contributor. I quickly called my friend LaTisha Bader PhD and asked her if she would take the project on with me. Dr. Bader is not only an amazing provider but she is a researcher who understands this subject inside and out. LaTisha and I spent the next three months putting together what would be a couple of pages in the book but was, as far as we know, the first published best practices for treating CUD. That chapter should help those of you working with patients presenting with CUD, and the book makes a great desk reference on other subjects.

I will start with the intake questions we use that help to paint a better picture of the individual. When you ask someone if they use any drugs you may often lose those who don't consider THC to be a drug or see it as medicine. I suggest specifically asking about their cannabis/THC use. Try, "Do you currently or have you recently used cannabis or THC in any form?" Just like the prior advice given to loved ones, the next step is to establish frequency, potency and method of ingestion. There is nothing really out of the ordinary in asking these questions but knowing the answers will help in building the patient profile. Get as specific as possible about the potency in particular; this will inform your treatment a great deal. Lastly we want to ask if they have a preference between indica or sativa. While the physiological differences are minor the answer may be telling. If someone only uses Indica they likely prefer a depressant effect, if Sativa the indication is more of an amphetamine perceived effect. If they say "either" or "doesn't matter" than they just want the intoxication and likely don't trend towards wanting to be high or laid out.

We are going to cover mental health effects separately but you may want to incorporate some of this into the intake questions. It is important to establish any potential mental illness that your patient may struggle with early on as it is most likely negatively impacted by their THC use. I begin by asking if there is a history of diagnosed mental health disorders. If they have been diagnosed in the past you can probe those symptoms alongside their use history to determine if it may be causal or if the use has worsened the symptoms.

In the majority of cases we treat the patient presents with mental health concerns. These can range from a bit of anxiety to audio and visual hallucinations. It is crucial that you treat the thought disorder(s) before getting into talk therapy with the individual; good luck talking about their childhood trauma if they believe they are under government or mafia surveillance! Assuming that there are symptoms of a mental health disorder your first order of business is to get a prescriber involved to treat those acute symptoms. This process can take time but can't really begin until abstinence has been established, the prescriber will have a much harder time treating symptoms if the patient continues to alter their brain chemistry with THC. I have seen this take any-where from a few days to several months and occasionally the determination is made that the issue is chronic not acute and the symptoms will have to be controlled with medication indefinitely. It is important to set expectations about this phase of treatment, since we don't know how long it will take to find a psychiatric baseline, so avoid suggesting a timeframe.

The next acute consideration is physical detox. While this is somewhat unpredictable you can typically expect to see worse symptoms in women than in men. Those symptoms peak around day 3 and there is a big resurgence of physical symptoms around the two week mark. Since THC is fat-soluble it stays in the system for a long time, out to 70 days in extreme cases. When the indi-vidual begins eating better and exercising regularly they will burn fat which will release THC back into their system. Be aware that you can see a spike in THC levels while the patient is detoxing even without use. This can trigger a positive drug test after several negatives depending on what your threshold for testing is.

Consult the DSM, page 518, for the full criteria and be pre-pared to deal with them.[2] I urge you to remember these symp-toms when treating in order to see them as the S&S of physical withdrawal as opposed to a noncompliant patient. We would nev-er consider a vomiting opiate addict who couldn't get out of bed to be noncompliant but since several of these S&S appear to be behavioral they can often be mistaken for a "bad attitude." As of this writing there is not an approved medication to treat THC PAWS, but two are in FDA phase two testing so expect them soon. In the absence of approved meds, prescribers try different things. I am not a prescriber, therefore I won't weigh in on these but will recommend aggressive hydration. This seems to help flush the system and encourage THC to move along as well as anything. If you have IV capabilities consider intravenous hydra-tion. One of the complications that will likely require IV hydra-tion is the presence of hyperemesis or cyclical vomiting. There is more being written on this relatively new phenomenon but much of it remains a mystery. Cannabis has long been understood to help with nausea, in fact the first approval of cannabis derived medications were for this purpose. We know that there are large concentrations of cannabinoid receptors in our digestive systems so the general thinking is that the unnaturally high levels of THC are for some reason having the opposite effect; rather than reducing nausea they are creating problems. Again, there are prescribers experimenting with medications to help with this but little is yet published more than specific case studies.

Having navigated through the acute phase, it is now time to treat the patient with CUD. While treatment is going to be the same as any other SUD, there are a few specific things for this patient that may help. Their road to treatment was likely a bit different than others. The patient with CUD may not enjoy the same support from their family or community as others do. For example, if a person asks for help quitting opiates, or alcohol or amphetamines the support for this effort is typically universal, everyone rallies around them, and oftentimes even their using peer group. The THC dependent individual is often met with skepticism from those around them who may hold antiquated beliefs that THC is not addictive or has never hurt anyone. These individuals are much less likely to support their recovery and may even play an active role in dissuading that recovery. Do not assume the same universal support for this individual as for others. For a multitude of reasons your patient's identity very well may revolve around their use. Their social circle and even their political circles often identify around their use of and support for THC. This substance enjoys a rather unique role in society today. Only alcohol is a more widely used intoxicant, yet everyone understands that even alcohol can be a problem for some and there is no debate about the other intoxicants. I have yet to see someone wearing a meth hat or heroin socks; people just think about weed differently. With this in mind, you want to make sure that you are safe and affirming and avoid all potential microaggressions. Comments like, "So it's just weed" "You believe you are addicted to marijuana" "You don't use any real drugs," can have a devastating effect on your patient. By the time they have made it to us they have typically run the gauntlet of people doubting them or questioning the severity of their addiction. They need to find support and encouragement in us. Depending on your specific line of work, keep in mind that there can be a hierarchy of drug use in recovery communities, especially in early recovery. People often want to trade war stories and establish which of them is the biggest baddest user. I have seen groups of addicts take jabs at the THC dependent patient, sometimes intentionally and sometimes unintentionally. Regardless of why, the behavior needs to be checked in the same way other glorification or downplaying of use is addressed.

One of the biggest differences with the CUD patient is helping them plan to engage in a world that is full of their Drug of Choice (DOC), with many references to their DOC, and with lots of misinformation and glorification of their DOC. There is also the recreational component. This differs a bit from many other substances but is somewhat similar to alcohol. For example, going to a concert or watching a movie may have been intertwined with their use for years and they have little or no history experiencing these things without THC. It's similar to the beer drinker who hasn't been to a sporting event in years without drinking being a part of the day. This often extends to eating. There are those who have not eaten regularly without the aid of THC, so we have to address this as well.

The final consideration is planning around the triggers they will be exposed to. Of all our senses, smell is the most triggering. Depending on where they live and what they do, the smell of weed growing, drying or burning may be a daily reality. There are places in Boulder and Denver where I can always count on at least one of those three and I prepare for it. It may be advisable for those in early recovery to do what they can to avoid the smell. If you are walking down a street with outdoor dining and people are drinking you won't smell their drinks but if you are anywhere near people smoking weed that smell will hit you.

There are also certain things like music or movies, even posters/wall hangings or decorations that might be triggering and will need to be discussed. Sometimes you will find that the CUD patient has a hard time identifying with certain kinds of music or other entertainment without their DOC. Addressing these potential triggers proactively can prevent a relapse.

I'd like to reiterate that treating CUD differs little from treating other substances; all we know about treating other drugs applies. What this chapter intends to do is provide additional, specific considerations.

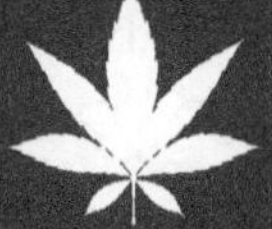

CHAPTER

15

TO THE USER

Thanks For Reading

So, somebody who loves you got you to agree to read this chapter or you are curious about "the other side" and picked it up on your own. Either way, I'm glad you are reading. I want to start by being perfectly clear, I don't know you or your situation and I respect you and your decisions, they are YOUR decisions. I am a recovering addict/alcoholic having taken my last drink/puff on 6/15/96. It has been a while since I have been there personally, but my life is filled with people thinking about or at the very beginning of their journey towards sobriety. I spend a great deal of time trying to better understand how and why people are using substances. I kind of focus on THC and what that use is doing in our brains and bodies. Very simply said, the majority of people who interact with cannabis will do so with few problems. I'm not here to convince you it's the 'devil's lettuce.' Equally and as simply; many people who interact with high THC potency weed or products will experience negative consequences from that use. Let me summarize a ton of science for you by saying that if you are using under 10% THC, not more than 3 times a month or so, and are over the age of 26 the chances of you having an issue with this substance are minimal. What the science tells us is that the further you are from those guidelines the greater the risk for harm. That means the further under the age of 26, the higher the THC potency, and the more frequently you use, the more potential for harm. Really simple math, don't complicate it!

I'll illustrate with two examples of use:

Thomas is 45 and smokes a joint or two every other weekend when he gets together with the guys. One of his buddies grows the weed and knows that it is about 10% THC and 3% CBD. Sidenote: I realize how tough it is to source weed at potency levels like this but it is out there, just mostly homegrown.

Ben is 19 and vapes a Pyramid Pen with 1g pods at 80% THC and 0 CBD. He hits the pen multiple times throughout the day and goes through a couple of cartridges a week.

In these scenarios I would have no concern for Thomas and great concern for Ben. The closer your use is to Ben's the more concerned I would be. So where does your use fall on that spectrum, more towards Thomas or more towards Ben?

Now that we have that little self assessment out of the way I am going to shift gears and talk to those of you who might or do have a problem with THC. First and foremost, welcome to the club! You are not even kind of remotely in any way alone with this struggle. Since weed has become as strong as it is today, there has been a huge uptick in people using in a way that is more harmful than helpful. What used to be a footnote in the addiction books is now causing about ⅓ of people who use at potency levels above 15% to develop a diagnosable addiction to THC. To this some of you are probably shaking your heads in disagreement and some are like 'Ya no shit, that's why I'm reading this.' Let me address the skeptic first. For years (like since the dawn of time) people could use weed and never develop a physical addiction to it. The only risk was a psychological addiction and potentially some negative cognitive effects, but those were pretty rare. In 2013 we were told by the scientists and doctors that THC could be physically addictive to a point where it would cause withdrawal for those who stopped.[1] If you have ever tried to quit or cut back you may have experienced some of these symptoms. Things like:

- Irritability/Anger/Aggression

- Nervousness or anxiety

- Sleep Difficulty (insomnia or disturbing dreams)

- Decreased appetite or weight loss

- Restlessness

- Depressed Mood

- Abdominal Pain, Shakiness/tremors, Sweating, Fever, Chills, Headache[2]

I want to be very clear here, 'weed' should not cause these issues, they are caused by consuming high potency THC. The thing that we need to keep in mind is how different these products are from the natural plant and get past the idea that "it's just weed." The farther above that 10% THC mark you are using the more likely you are to have some issues, which can range from pretty minor to extremely serious. For those of you who will swear up and down that you don't have a problem, all I ask is that you recognize that some people (increasing in number) do have a problem with THC. By recognizing that it is possible we can have a much more honest dialogue with ourselves and be more helpful to others. Remember, you don't have to convince me of anything, I am writing to help those who do or may have an issue. If that's not you, fantastic; but I hope you will continue reading. The easiest way to prove to yourself and those who care about you that it's not a problem is simply to take a month off. Pick a day, tell someone what you're doing and give yourself a tolerance reset of 30 days. If you can pull that off without much trouble odds are you haven't crossed a line.

Now to those of you who know that something isn't right with your use. Maybe you have tried to stop and been unable. Maybe your mental health is struggling and you find yourself with anxiety that gets worse when you add THC. Maybe your physical health is in decline and you are having trouble eating or keeping food down. Maybe it has gotten as serious as being unable to control painful vomiting that is only relieved by super hot showers. Whatever the case is, you know or suspect that your use may be getting in the way of life. I think the easiest way to think about it is that maybe you are not being served by the substance anymore and you might be serving it. If you are anything like me, it's a really complicated feeling that is lonely and feels pretty damn hopeless. I knew that my use was causing problems but I couldn't imagine stopping. There was a part of me that wanted to at least take a break, but a bigger part warned me that doing so would be a mistake. I was able to remember and reference the good times but was having more and more trouble repeating them. I wasn't getting high with people and having fun, I was just using to feel normal. One of the hardest things for me was that I had nothing in common with people who didn't use/drink, but I was feeling more and more disconnected from those who did. It seemed like some of them were still having fun and I was on the outside. One of my best friends sums it up so well. He says that our tendency is to think about and remember our use as a business ledger, but we only look at the money coming in and not the expenses. If you look at the books for my business and only look at what we earn you'd expect me to be loaded! But when you look at all we spend, you see the real story, we stay afloat. Every set of books has two sides, the ins and the outs. If the "outs" associated with your life while using are greater than the "ins" it might be time to take a look at things.

At this point I think the hardest thing for me was to realize that I wasn't a victim, what I was experiencing wasn't just because of stuff other people did; most of it was a direct result of my actions. I just kept saying that it wasn't fair rather than look at it all and consider what people were telling me. One of the hardest things you will ever do is to take a step back and consider what people are telling you and to ask yourself a few, really tough questions; "Am I living the life I want? Am I moving towards a place where I want to be? And if not, is THC getting in the way?" Even if the answer to that last one is, "I don't know, maybe," I encourage you to make a change. I'm going to ask you to stop using; not just THC but anything that will alter your mood. It's no use quitting one thing just to use another in the same way for the same reasons. The reality is that if nothing changes then everything will stay the same! You have nothing to lose by stopping for a bit and then asking yourself which of the two lives you like more. What I found was that while quitting was the hardest thing I had ever done, it turned out to be the best decision of my life. Today I don't abstain because I have to, I do because I want to. Well, at least most days I want to. On the days I don't, I remember what it was like and then try to "play the movie out" as we say in the 12-step world. What happens after I pick up again: that day, that month, the future? I have to remember to think past just the moment of getting high. While I won't lie and say it's easy and everything after is simple and awesome, I will tell you that

I wouldn't trade the clarity and the relationships I have now for anything. Being substance free has allowed me to live my best life. Not an easy life, or a simple one, but the best I could hope for.

If you want to give it a shot, see what it's like on the other side, or just to prove that you can, I have a few suggestions that might help.

- Pick your start date carefully. You are going to be doing something that will likely be pretty tough and you don't want to do it the day before starting a new job or something like that. I suggest you pick the first day of a "weekend" or whenever you will have a couple of days free.

- Have your last use be afternoon/evening. This will give you a good chunk of time (sleeping hopefully) to start off. For most people that first and second day are some of the hardest, so let's do all we can to get through them.

- Expect some level of withdrawal. Many of the suggestions that follow will help with that, but expecting it can help. While it is different for everyone, you can probably expect it to get rough at the end of day 2 and day 3 will be when your body really starts to demand you add THC. It's going to communicate this in the ways I mentioned above so be ready for it.

- Stock up on stuff that you like to eat. There are no restrictions on diet during this time. We just want you to be getting calories and those come easier in foods you love. Give yourself several days of good meals and plenty of snacks.

- Hydrate! This may sound like generic, basic advice that everyone gives but it's super important for you at this time. Avoid sodas for this, those fall under snacks, drink lots of water and sports drinks. Lots!

- Build a schedule that is pretty tight at the beginning then chills out, taking you out to a month. The first 3 days you really want to be taking it easy, ideally you will exercise some. If exercise isn't a part of your life right now then try to get up and walk for 30 minutes twice a day. In addition to building exercise in, make sure to include recreation, schedule things you like to do. You also want to schedule seeing people if that is helpful and ideally seeing people who can help you with this process. By the time your month's schedule is done you should have one or two things to look forward to every day if possible.

- Avoid triggers. Don't stop three days before going to the Pink Floyd light show at your local planetarium or whatever. If there is a concert scheduled that you know will be hard not to use, you need to avoid that show. Plan it out so you aren't going to be in places where people are using. Is there music you need to avoid for a bit, things that might get you thinking about weed too much? What about entertainment? I wouldn't suggest watching Friday or Dazed and Confused for a bit. Give yourself a break from seeing people use. Of all our senses smell is the one that hits us the hardest, so avoid being in places where you will smell weed.

- Tell at least one person what you're doing. You will want support at some point, someone to reach out too, establish that before starting.

- Keep a daily journal; please trust me on this one. It doesn't have to be a big deal, but it's important. All you need to do is write a minimum of 3 words every day and it doesn't have to have anything to do with this. Not only do you never need to show this to someone, it's best if you don't. This exercise is for you alone, something to look back on if needed.

- Don't give up. I absolutely believe that you can stop but if you have trouble and slip up instead of saying, "Screw it," just start again. This is where that journal might be nice. Pick another start day and get back after it. Consider adding some more resources this time, would a professional or someone in recovery be helpful?

If quitting on your own proves tough please consider getting some help with it. There are self help groups (Marijuana Anonymous) and plenty of good professionals out there at multiple levels of care.

I'm going to close this out in the same way I started, I don't know you or your situation. What I do know is that for many of us this struggle is very real and despite how hard it is I've never met a person who wanted it who wasn't able to make the change. You might need additional support but you can do this. If it wasn't better for me on this side of things I wouldn't be out there encouraging people to try living sober. It absolutely won't solve all of life's problems but often it helps to shed a few and lets you focus more on solutions for the others.

Above all, keep fighting for it. There is a saying in the recovery world, "The miracle you are looking for is in the work you don't want to do. Don't stop before the miracle has a chance."

CHAPTER 16

WOMEN AND WEED

Introducing Dr. Latisha Bader

D r Bader is one of the best clinicians I have ever met let alone had the privilege to work alongside. She is my go-too person for lots of stuff, but especially on the topic of female physiology and THC. A little while back I was asked to give a talk to a group in Montana, composed of moms in recovery and those who treat them. They asked me to explain the effects of *in utero* and early childhood exposure. My first call was to LaTisha. She directed me to relevant research and recounted a lot of what she sees in her daily life; she treats women.

Although I talk and write about THC all the time, what I found in researching the subject made me more emotional than I have been about anything related to this subject in a very long time. The data told stories of women often picking THC over the well-being of their children. Protecting our offspring is one of the strongest biological pulls that we have, but THC was proving stronger for many. Behind the data were the lives of individual moms and kids, that reality made for some very emotional research.

I couldn't write this book without a dedicated section to understanding the differences in male/female THC use and I don't think there is a better person anywhere to unpack it than my brilliant and dear friend Dr. LaTisha Bader…. Clap, you should all be clapping now, even if you're alone; put 'em together!

Women and Weed

It's not always the same

When people are having difficulty seeing the perspective of another person, I get out a coin. I position the two parties across from each other and ask them to take note of what they see and what they believe for about 30 seconds. Then I invite them to argue their point of view. I find that people become very talkative, get a bit impassioned, then develop a loyalty to the principle of not changing their perspective. It can get a little loud and a little heated. Then I turn the coin on its side. With the lesson that they are usually arguing the same concept, just with a one-sided perspective. And ask if they would be willing to see a different side.

I hold this belief when it comes to treatment, substances, policy, and life. If you only know one side of the coin, you don't have a grasp of the entire situation. Taking the time to flip over the coin and learn something new, adds dimension to your understanding and possibly some compassion

Cannabis is no different. It seems historically, like with many other mind-mood altering substances, we have placed ourselves on one side or the other and are arguing. As I joined the conversation and the treatment of cannabis, it was evident that cannabis use was quickly becoming a very different reality depending on who was using and how they were using. The consequences of use for adolescents vs. adults, pets vs. people, and edibles vs. dabbing are quite distinct. One of the nuances that promptly became apparent to me was that there were vast gender differences. I started to use a phrase to depict a simple, yet pivotal fact – *substances are gender inclusive, but they are NOT gender neutral, especially when it came to cannabis.*

As a licensed psychologist, licensed addiction counselor and certified mental performance consultant, I had been involved in treating individuals with substance use disorders for the better part of 20 years. I wasn't surprised by the impact of substance use on our bodies as professionals, athletes and women. But as I served as Chief Clinical Officer at Women's Recovery, a gender-specific Intense Outpatient Program (IOP), I was continuously alarmed at the impact I was seeing when people were using cannabis. I presented my first "Women and Weed" talk in 2018 and haven't stopped since. Because of biological, psychological, and social reasons, when women use, the impact is exponentially worse.

Historical knowledge of gender differences

There was a concept that began in medical training in the 80's labeled the telescoping effect that illustrated that substances had a greater impact on female bodies. With the support of a few studies

(Piazza et al 1986; Piazza, Vrbka, & Yeager 1989; SAMSHA 2009; Becker, McClellan & Glover Reed, 2017; TIPS 51), the concept was introduced but did not get much traction. The popularity and understanding of gender differences in substance use hasn't grown much since that time, but the impacts are significant. A limited amount of substance use research is dedicated to the understanding of women's issues, and only since the 1990's have women even been part of the research population (NIH 2001; Clayton & Collins 2014; NIDA 2021). Women weren't included in research because 1) they were more biologically complicated than men, and 2) as primary caregivers of young children, women had too many competing demands to participate in research (National Bioethics Committee 2001). So, because of this historical indifference, it's worth taking a few pages to describe how cannabis might be a different journey for women.

To highlight the telescoping effect, essentially women have the "same disease at different rates." Women will typically start with lower levels of substance use, but end up escalating use to a higher degree of use and dependence. Because of differences in body composition 1) higher fat content, 2) lower volume of water, and 3) less gastric enzymes, female bodies process substances at different rates and in different ways.

Women also use for different reasons. Studies confirm that women use for mood regulation and stress reduction over risk taking. (TIP 51; NIH 2020; SAMSHA 2022). NIH (2020) suggesting the top four reasons for substance use are fighting exhaustion, coping with pain, self-treating mental health problems, and controlling weight.

Cannabis intoxication also occurs in different places in the body with differing effects. Gender differences in the endocannabinoid system have been found in numerous studies. Even the industry suggests sex differences in the effects of cannabis use; men experience lower body temperatures, greater increase in appetite and less sensitivity to pain relief while women are more likely to get dizzy, have decrease in gastric motility and stimulated sex organs (Blanton et al 2021).

Cravings and urges have also been reported to be more severe for women (DSM 5 2013). Cannabis withdrawal has been documented (DSM-5 TR; Hermann, Weerts & Vandrey 2015) to be about twice as hard for women. Between body functioning and the fact that cannabis is a fat-soluble (lipophilic) drug (vs. water soluble drug like alcohol and nicotine) women find withdrawal symptoms more intense.

Through the process of beginning, using and cessation of cannabis it is just *different* for women. Although it has been marketed as a cure all, literally more than 30 ailments depending on which state's medical card registry you reference, the adverse impacts for women haven't been highlighted.

Marketing Cannabis

If we turn our attention to how substances are introduced, culture and marketing illustrate a predictable development. The interesting thing about the relationship between women and substances often comes before we ever try them. History repeats the lesson that when a substance is initially marketed, instead of marketing to women; women ARE the marketing.

Figure 2: *Yasmin L. Hurd 1* , Jacqueline-Marie N. Ferland 1 , Yoko Nomura 1,2,3,4 , Leslie A. Hulvershorn 5 , Kevin M.Gray6 andChristianThurstone7*

Figure 3: Canadian Centre on Substance Abuse

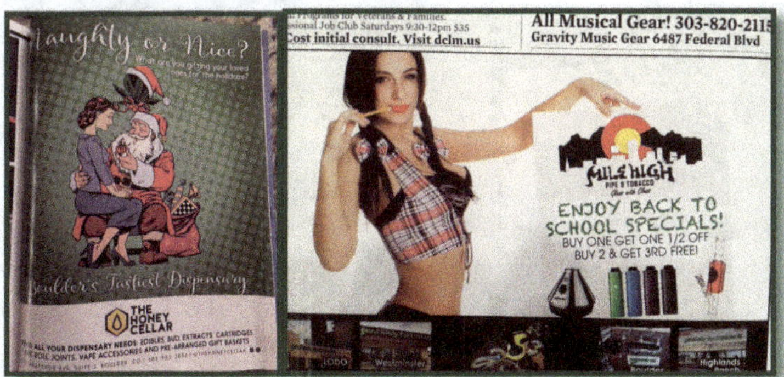

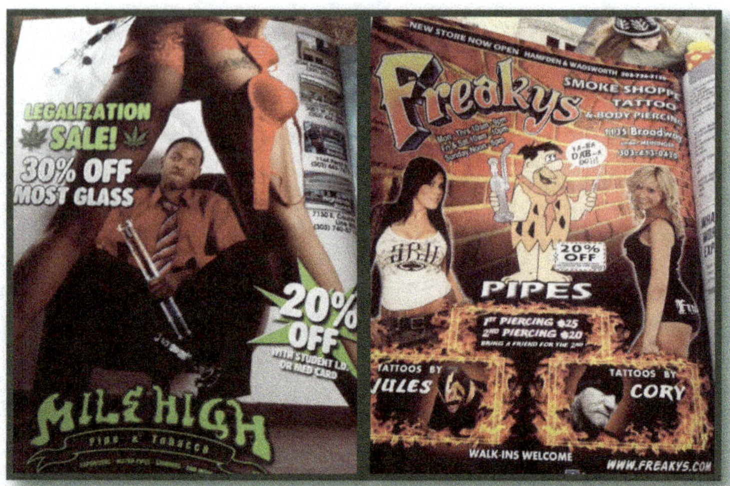
LEGALIZATION SALE!
30% OFF MOST GLASS
20% OFF
WITH STUDENT I.D. OR RED CARD
MILE HIGH
PIPE & TOBACCO

NEW STORE NOW OPEN   HAMPDEN & WADSWORTH
Freakys
SMOKE SHOPPE
TATTOO
& BODY PIERCING
1935 Broadway
20% OFF
PIPES
1ST PIERCING $25
2ND PIERCING $20
BRING A FRIEND FOR THE 2ND
TATTOOS BY JULES
TATTOOS BY CORY
WALK-INS WELCOME
WWW.FREAKYS.COM

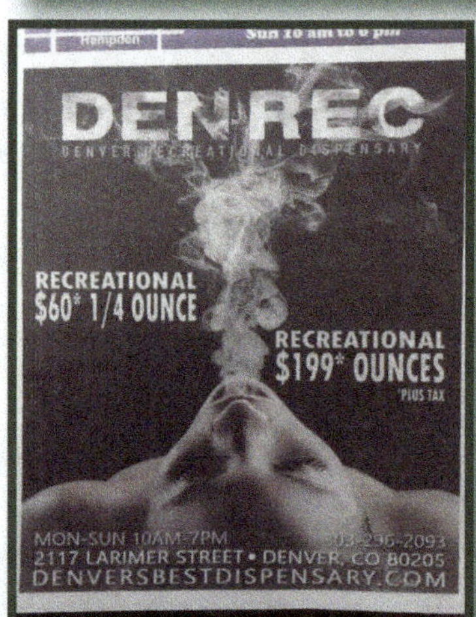
Hampden   Sun 10 am to 6 pm
DENREC
DENVER RECREATIONAL DISPENSARY
RECREATIONAL $60* 1/4 OUNCE
RECREATIONAL $199* OUNCES
*PLUS TAX
MON-SUN 10AM-7PM   303-295-2093
2117 LARIMER STREET • DENVER, CO 80205
DENVERSBESTDISPENSARY.COM

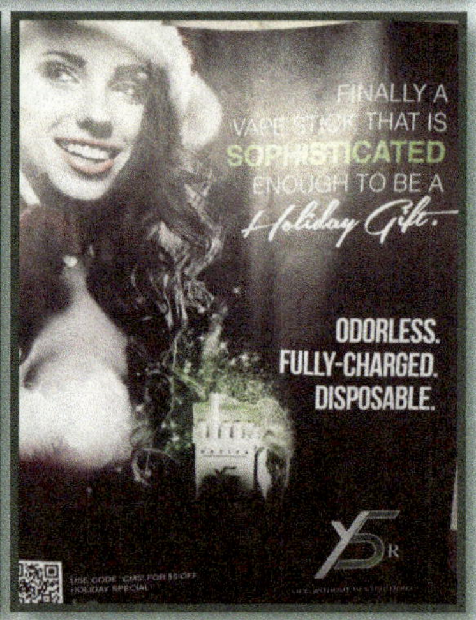
FINALLY A VAPE STICK THAT IS
SOPHISTICATED
ENOUGH TO BE A
Holiday Gift.
ODORLESS.
FULLY-CHARGED.
DISPOSABLE.
USE CODE "GMS" FOR $5 OFF
HOLIDAY SPECIAL
Y5R

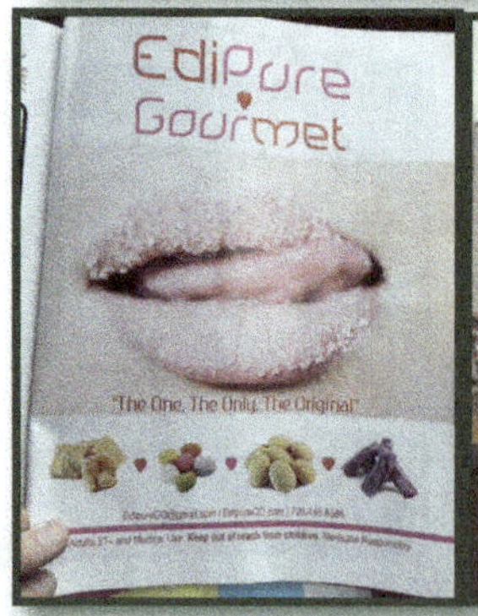
EdiPure
Gourmet
"The One, The Only, The Original"

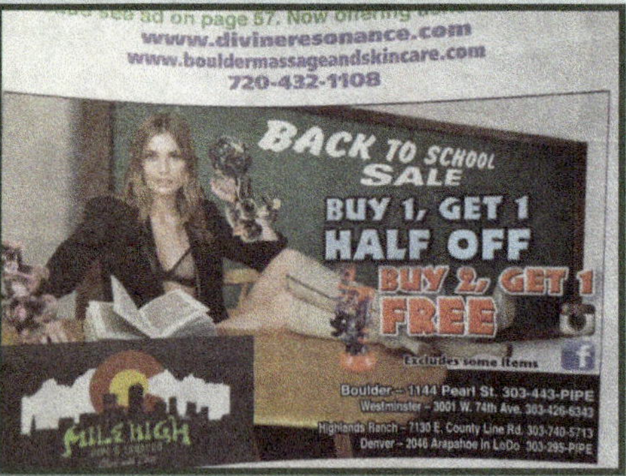
see ad on page 57. Now offering
www.divineresonance.com
www.bouldermassageandskincare.com
720-432-1108
BACK TO SCHOOL SALE
BUY 1, GET 1 HALF OFF
BUY 2, GET 1 FREE
Excludes some items
Boulder – 1144 Pearl St. 303-443-PIPE
Westminster – 3001 W. 74th Ave. 303-426-6343
Highlands Ranch – 7130 E. County Line Rd. 303-740-5713
Denver – 2046 Arapahoe in LoDo 303-295-PIPE
MILE HIGH

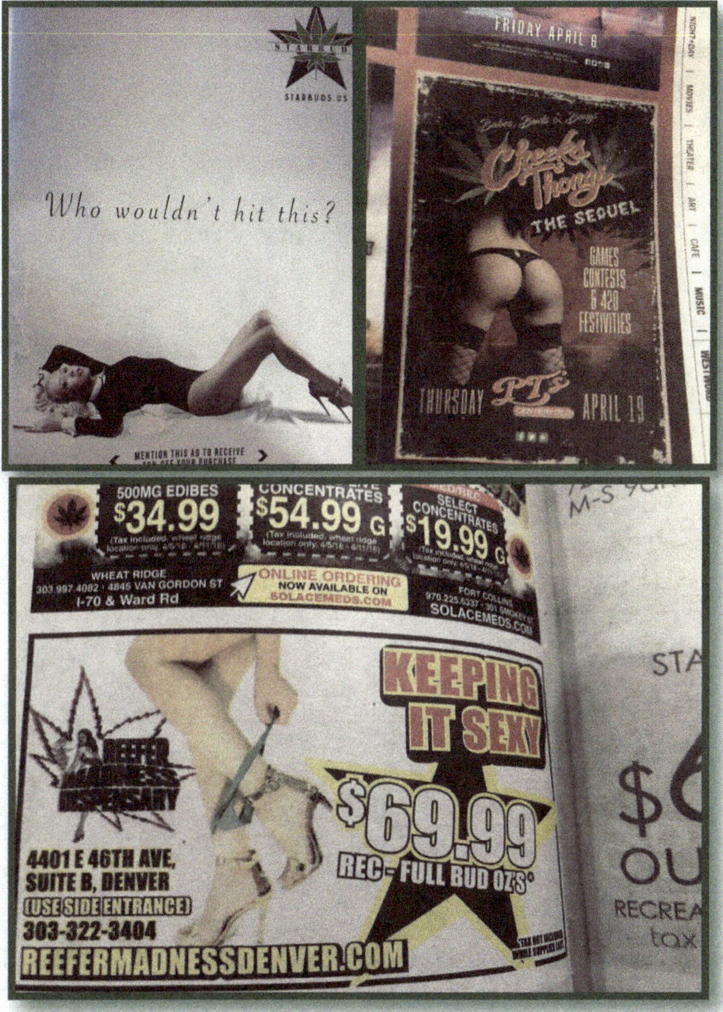

When cannabis was first legalized, the advertisements were that *of* women. Between buxom coeds, cartoon characters and center fold layouts with marketing tags of "Who wouldn't hit this?" One could recognize that women were not the initial target audience. The same conversion can be seen over the generations with other industries such as tobacco and alcohol, remember the Budweiser girls?

With this quick flood of ads, the industry secured the first wave of new users, mostly young men. Then they continued to pour their energy into getting additional new users, making recreational users into regular users, and then transforming those regular users into chronic users. The industry increased the potency, invented countless products and continued to decrease the perceived risk of THC use while skyrocketing the intensity of products. Once this initial market was secured, they moved on.

Around 2017, I noticed a push to bring women into the market. The marketing campaigns pivoted and the depiction of a cannabis user had moved from a sultry co-ed over to models who would have been at home in Cosmopolitan with tag lines of "9 Reasons Why Weed is Made for Women." If you spent time engaging in internet research or perusing social media algorithms, you could have concluded that cannabis could relieve anxiety and stress, improve your sex life, help with weight maintenance, get high faster than men, alleviate PMS symptoms, prevent and treat cancer, alleviate pregnancy symptoms and help you enjoy life. Even as an educated consumer and treatment provider, I had to admit the promises sounded glorious.

I once heard that if a medicine or supplement could treat more than three physical or psychological concerns in the same product, you should be very skeptical. For example, if Tylenol, could decrease knee pain, reduce a fever and sky rocket your libido, you might want to question the veracity of those claims. But the marketing continued to tout cannabis' vast ability to accomplish many promises for our health and well-being. This advice to remain skeptical, and the ever-increasing research led me to question the claims that were being made because they just didn't line up.

Marketing included a strong message about pain relief of many kinds - physical, mental and emotional. It was publicized for being safe at all stages of life, for children, during pregnancy and for the elderly.

One hallmark marketing campaign from the industry, which was followed up by survey to quantify the actual number of times it occurred, found that 83% of the medical dispensaries suggested cannabis use for pregnant women (National Survey on Drug Use and Health 2018; Dickson et al 2018). The recommendations were being made by budtenders based on personal opinion and instructions from dispensaries to endorse the use of cannabis throughout a woman's pregnancy; often sharing that it was safe and that there was little impact on the fetus. Cannabis *is* able to decrease nausea, not a new fact about the plant, which is why it was being positioned as a treatment for symptoms of pregnancy. The industry's message was changing the behaviors of women at a record pace. There were studies that documented increased use of THC during pregnancy. Pregnant women (15-44) reported 108% increase in monthly use in 3 years (2015 to 2018). Cannabis was the most common illicit drug used during pregnancy, with rates as high as 30% (Gunn 2015; NSDUH 2019; Brown et al 2017; Volkow 2019).

I wasn't stunned when I saw a marketing strategy that was targeting directly to women and heavily researched – sex (Lynn 2019). CB1 receptors are all over our bodies including a cluster of them located in and around female genitalia. When any product or substance can make those receptors tingle or provide increased sensitivity you are more likely to achieve orgasm. Those "tingly lady bits" appeared to be a great money maker for the industry.

What fails to get discussed is that an impairing substance is now being used to disrupt the brain and connectivity in order to achieve a different physical state. In a reductionist view, I need to get high to have sex. Although it helps me say "yes" and maybe achieve orgasm, it places a barrier between me and my partner and can cause significant changes in my ability to consent and stay safe. It is a story that goes back in time to figure out how to juggle being vulnerable, intimate, combat negative self-talk, quiet messages of body shame, address attachment, all the while keeping the body performing. Sex is never simple. And many people choose to use substances in order to be intimate. (In no way is that just a female concern).

We can move now to the next marketing messages of "cana-parenting" and how cannabis can help us be more relaxed and well-grounded people. This recycled message was used by pharmaceutical companies who suggested that we could achieve better patience and parenting with "mommy's little helpers." Barbiturates, benzodiazepines and booze have all been positioned in front of parents in order to take the edge off of parenting stress.

In the children's book by Wendy Brazill called *When Mommy Gets High (2021)*, an explanation for why parents might retreat into another room to use and then return with a restored sense of calm, illustrates why cannabis could better us as parents. What we know is that putting a chemical barrier of any kind between you and another person, doesn't have a lasting positive effect. It was being marketed as a good parenting practice, and this was really difficult for me to digest as a treatment provider for moms.

Inclusively, the marketing messages to women highlighted pleasure, aesthetics, culture, curing cancer, entrepreneurship, eco-friendly innovation, and holistic approaches to self-care and profit. But the loudest messages, that were in bold print in magazines, books and dispensary commercials, were going to be the progressive impact on mental and physical health. Messages suggested that cannabis use was going to treat mental health and help women find their "higher self."

Impact on the Mind and Body

THC is the number one illicit drug used by women, with 14.8% or 21,000,000 women using it in the past year, reflecting a significant increase from the year before (SAMSHA 2019). There will be little surprise when this number continues to climb year after year.

Back to the telescoping affect, with the female body having a different composition of fat, water, and hormones cannabis has distinctive impacts. One noticeable difference comes early in puberty. Cannabis can cause changes to the menstrual cycle (delaying or inhibiting ovulation) (Ilnitsky & Uum 2019). With these hormonal disruptions, girls and women can experience a direct impact on their physical development and overall health, much less fertility. Knowing that women use for mood regulation (NIH 2020), it was easy to forecast that experimentation or recreation use would turn into more.

Studies confirm that recreational use of cannabis is turning into regular use and then to chronic use at startling rates. It's now suggested that 30% of cannabis users meet criteria for a cannabis use disorder. This number has increased from 11% to 30% in about 8 years. (Leung et al 2020).

To those outside of the field these numbers might seem considerable, but to those in the field they are alarming. In essence that means that cannabis has moved from addiction rates similar to alcohol to that of nicotine, a highly addictive substance. With a quick reminder that cannabis withdrawal is more difficult for women.

In conjunction with the physical, there's also the emotional and interpersonal impacts. In the Journal of Experimental and Clinical Pharmacology, MacKenzie and Cservenka (2021) report how the use of cannabis impacts our emotional systems. They suggested that the use of cannabis decreases emotional regulation and influences emotional processing, observing that THC increases anxiety in fearful situations. But the most impactful finding was the reduced ability to identify emotions. In particular, there was decreased accuracy and response time to identify <u>happiness, sadness or anger</u>.

When I step back and think about the basic emotions needed to communicate, these are imperative. With attunement to these feelings, I have the ability to discern the fundamental aspects of a parent-child relationship. "Is mom happy? Is dad sad?" The study goes on to report that without this attunement there is a weakening of interpersonal relationships and increasing emotional distress. These findings were not at all surprising, they just made the family stories I have heard and the times spent treating cannabis use disorders that much clearer. The emotional message wasn't getting through.

Up to this point in a woman's life, you could conceptualize that substance use has a more of a direct impact on herself as well as some on others. But no period could be as impactful as that during pregnancy.

I heard a quote once that suggested that the *truth* was often very quiet in comparison to how loud the rest of a marketing message could be. One needed to listen for the quiet truth. This seems like the facts when it comes to women's health. There is an overabundance of reputable, evidence-based science that confirms that cannabis use during pregnancy is unsafe and yet the messaging from the scientific community wasn't as loud as that of the industry. The reality was clear and the facts were present to those who were treating women who were using during pregnancy – the outcomes are not good.

In 2019 The Surgeon General VADM Jerome Adams, made a statement that "No amount of marijuana use during pregnancy is known to be safe." I know, sometimes it feels small, but statements like these are many years in the making. In order to get black box warnings, public service announcements (PSA) on posters that are placed in bathrooms, or statements from government officials take time, outcomes, deaths, and surmounting evidence-based studies.

General acceptance of warnings, like this, often take years or decades after a public health statement is first made. Consider alcohol use and pregnancy, tobacco use and pregnancy, pharmaceuticals and pregnancy; these adverse outcomes took decades to be accepted by the general population while the medical field was already treating Fetal Alcohol Syndrome and placing babies in the NICU for low birth weight due to nicotine use for decades. Today they are recognized as indisputable facts.

Politically, it can also take years of litigation and billions of dollars to reverse a belief and confirm something has a negative impact on our health. Think about processed foods, asbestos, lead in paint, or even pollution. Then consider that, for women, there is a critical period of life during reproductive years that small exposures to somewhat "benign" foods, medications and environmental toxins can have momentous impacts on our reproductive health and development of a child. Medical providers did not have an approach to best practices and many women were getting recommendations from budtenders and personal recommendations instead (Barbosa-Leiker et al 2021; Celestina et al 2021; Peiper et al 2017; Haug et al 2016, Dickson et al 2018; Forray et al 2015).

Reports suggest it is the most widely used illicit substance used during pregnancy with up to 30% endorsing use (SAMSHA 2019). 18.1% of pregnant women who were using cannabis in the past year met the criteria for cannabis use disorder. Nearly ½ of women who regularly smoke cannabis continue to use during pregnancy. In one study, 7.1% of pregnant women (ages 15-44) reported using in the past month. And daily use increased from 1.2% to 3.1% in a 2-year period (108% increase) (SAMSHA, 2019; NSDUH, 2016; Gunn et al 2016; Bailey, Wood & Shah 2020; Ko et al, 2015).

What I don't think is clearly known or communicated, is that cannabis freely crosses the placenta and exposes the fetus. There is no protection between the mother and the developing child and cannabis can reach high concentrations for the fetus with repeated exposure.

It's been suggested that once a woman learns she is pregnant it takes on average 4 months to establish and maintain sobriety. Getting sober is a difficult process but one that women might choose if faced with accurate information about the risks or hazards of a substance or behavior.

Studies suggest the reasons for use during pregnancy are to relieve stress, nausea / vomiting, pain, to have fun and relax, and relieve symptoms of a chronic condition (Ko et al 2017; Besse, Parikh & Mark 2023). "We know that cannabinoid signaling plays a role in modulating stress, which is why some people use cannabis to reduce anxiety and relax," said Yoko Nomura, Professor of Psychology at CUNY Graduate Center and Queens College. "But our study shows that *in utero* exposure to cannabis has the opposite effect on children, causing them to have increased levels of anxiety, aggression, and hyperactivity compared to other children who were not exposed to cannabis during pregnancy." (Rompala, Nomura & Hurd 2021).

There is a basic understanding that exposure to chemicals on our developing brain during utero can have lasting effects, called epigenetics. They can turn on/off the receptors that impact the overall development of a brain. If a woman decides to use cannabis during any portion of her pregnancy the following impacts may occur. As early as 5 weeks into gestation, the endocannabinoid system (ECS) can be detected in the fetus. Since THC disrupts the mothers ECS it also impacts the fetus. CB1 receptors are expressed differently in the fetal brain and the use of cannabis during pregnancy can disrupt the sequential pattern of normal neuronal development. This early disruption can lead to numerous impacts later in life.

A significant concern for cannabis use during pregnancy revolves around the rates of low birth weight. Marijuana exposure to newborns in utero had worse outcomes than the control group: weighing less, more likely to be pre-term or admitted to the NICU (Bailey, Wood & Shah 2020; Gunn et al 2016). Reports also suggest smaller head circumference. (Dodge et al 2023). These results were increased if a mother uses it throughout pregnancy versus the third trimester. Children who are born with low birth weight and smaller head circumference are more at risk for poorer health outcomes (i.e., depression, social dysfunction, developmental conditions like ADHD and cognitive delay, and increased risk for chronic diseases as adults).

Women can have increased rates of anemia, and precipitous labor. Marijuana use during pregnancy is associated with 2.3 times greater stillbirth. (National Institutes of Health 2013; Dodge et al 2023; Drug Lactation Database).

At birth, the concerns continue. Neonatal Abstinence Syndrome (also called NAS) is a group of conditions caused when a baby withdraws from certain drugs they are exposed to in the womb before birth. Smoking THC reduces the amount of oxygen in fetal blood similar to smoking tobacco. Infants of mothers who use drugs (including cannabis) and/or alcohol during their pregnancy may experience a withdrawal process in the days following birth. Neonatal withdrawal from cannabis includes poorer feeding, poorer tone, hypertonicity, irritability and infant toxicity (Jones & Felder 2015; Pan & Yi 2013).

Mothers also have their own struggles post-partum. Increase in cannabis use often occurs after delivery. Women return to use following pregnancy to treat symptoms of postpartum or return to use because the perceived risk has passed. (Davis et al 2020; Wymore et al 2021; Joyce, Thompson & Good 2021)

If cannabis use starts, returns or continues after childbirth and the mother chooses to breastfeed the risks endure. THC crosses into breast milk (lipophilic). It can accumulate to high concentrations (8 times higher than maternal plasma) and can be found in breastmilk as quickly as 1 hour and last up to 6 weeks. (Davis et al 2020; Wymore et al 2021; Garner et al 2022). Breastfeeding with milk that contains THC can have cognitive, social, and motor effects on the child both with short term and long-term effects.

Research shows that children exposed to THC in utero and through breast milk can show gaps in problem solving and memory at school, more irritability and trembling as an infant, have decreased motor development at 12 months, and develop inattention and hyperactivity in childhood. Children whose mothers used marijuana during pregnancy were 50% more likely to be diagnosed with autism (Miller et al 2023).

Data from the CDC, reflects that there has been a 49% increase in pediatric cancer rates from 1975 to 2015. Cannabis was shown to be spatiotemporal and casually related to the rise in pediatric cancers. THC and cannabigerol (CBG) were a cause of pediatric cancers (Reece and Hulse 2021; Reece and Hulse 2021). Acute Lymphoid Leukemia (ALL) is the most common childhood cancer whose incidence rose 93.51% in 20 years. The researchers used data from the CDC, the National Cancer Institute and the National Survey on Drug Use and Health showing that cannabis consumption is associated with ALL and satisfied the criteria for causality.

During early childhood development the impacts of neonatal cannabis exposure can be seen in the home, classroom and interpersonally. Lower scores on verbal reasoning and memory tasks, poor language comprehension, visual and perceptual functions were reported. Deficits are seen in impulse control, problem-solving, attention span, and analytical skills among older children. Lower global achievement, reading, spelling and math scores were also reported (Adolescent Brain Cognitive Development; Miller et al 2023).

Study results suggest problems with neurological development (hyperactivity, aggression, poor cognitive functioning, stress sensitivity, changes in dopaminergic receptors, and increases in diagnosis of autism and ADHD). Additionally, there were increased risks for pathology in middle childhood (psychotic-like experiences, depression, anxiety, impulsivity, attention, social problems and sleep disturbance) (Miller et al 2023; Rompala, Nomura & Hurd 2021).

As science catches up with the reality of neonatal exposure to cannabis, the findings continue to mount suggesting that there are significant risks associated with use, but this hasn't seemed to deter use. The Colorado Department of Public Health and Environment, Pregnancy Assessment Monitoring System (PRAMS) data from 2014-2019 suggested increased rates of use in *all* categories - before pregnancy, during pregnancy, postpartum, and postpartum currently breastfeeding.

Because of the adverse effects to the developing fetus and infant brains, the Society of Obstetricians and Gynecologists of

Canada (2022; Grave et al 2022) and America (2017) recommend that all pregnant and breastfeeding women abstain from marijuana use. This represents a substantial period of time that a woman might want to make different choices for the health of herself, and her family.

Once this critical period of life comes to a close and women continue to age, there are more opportunities to market and use cannabis. During premenopausal, perimenopause and menopause, and post menopause cannabis has become a recommended supplement for symptom relief, hormonal balance, as an anxiolytic, and anti-inflammatory.

In a survey of women 35 and over, where participants reported current cannabis use, they endorsed using cannabis for menopause-related symptoms (78.7%) Most common reasons for current use were sleep (65%), anxiety (45%) and muscle/joint achiness (33%). (Joyce et al 2021; Babyn et al 2023). Discomfort with joint pain, memory changes, sleep disturbance, hormone imbalance, and a decrease in cognitive acuity have all been reasons to try cannabis with little science about the impact.

If you are still reading, thanks! I hope that skimming the surface of the science pertaining to women's bodies, health and families suggests that this topic isn't one to shy away from. Cannabis use can be introduced anytime during the lifespan, with some stages having significantly more impact and consequence. It might sound alarmist, but we really are changing generations. The substantial influence of cannabis on a women's body, family and home represent reason enough to continue to research and share specific gender differences. Cannabis is being positioned as a solution in a woman's world, and it only represents one side of the coin.

I hope that this small change in perspective can represent a new way of considering the impact of any substance or behavior. Sometimes there isn't a level playing field, even when it comes to substances.

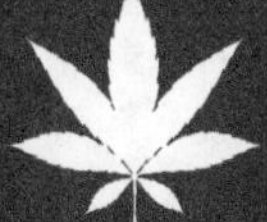

CHAPTER

17

MY CRYSTAL BALL(S)

What to Expect Next

Remember that children's book "If You Give A Mouse A Cookie?" If not, the plot is pretty simple. A child gives a cookie to a mouse and ends up having a grand party at the house because the mouse wanted a glass of milk to go with its cookie and so on.[1] One of the descriptions of the book I found online sums it up nicely : "Each event that occurs makes the mouse want something new, creating a seemingly endless stream of demands."[2]

The weed predicament in the country is like that book; the cookie was Amendment 64 in Colorado. What started with products sold in a well regulated industry, where communities could opt out and nothing would change except for losing tax dollars, has taken off in ways no one anticipated.

That's because, once the weed industry had their cookie (recreational sales), the demands for more grew and grew. The first demand was a coordinated effort to overturn the retail bans many communities had in place. It wasn't enough to have retail, the guys who owned that retail wanted to expand their market and have more retail. The problem was that a community had to defeat every single challenge and the industry had to only win once. They could win in several ways too, like in Longmont, Colorado. The weed proponents got the city council to approve retail sales, even though the community voted it down twice. This idea even went so far as to see a bill introduced in the state of California that would require a certain number of dispensaries in all communities. The idea behind it was that if the community said, "no," the industry would get to set up retail because obviously they know what's best for the community.[3] In one of the shadiest examples of industry being in bed with local leadership, the town of Hancock Maryland allowed a multistate operator (now owned by Trulive) to open up shop in town in exchange for a 5% take of the companies profits. The two parties are of course now in arbitration because they are disagreeing on what a "profit" is.[4] Money and manipulation have always been powerful motivators.

Now with the immense wealth these companies have amassed, they can afford to do what it really takes to change laws in America and that is of course hire high powered lawyers to complain and sue over anything that is getting in the way of profits. While there are endless examples of this taking place on everything from pushing back established boundaries with schools and churches to making sure nobody can limit THC potency, one of the best examples is how companies are now throwing a fit about the miniscule amount of testing of their products that is actually taking place is in Oregon. A law was passed there requiring that the weed sold in their 'tightly regulated market' adhere to some pretty basic public safety issues, such as restrictions on allowing for large concentrations of Fungus Aspergillus.[5] That law hit the books and immediately The Cannabis Industry Association of Oregon led a lawsuit to reverse the law. Since infection from this fungus can cause things like coughing up blood and shortness of breath, it made good medical sense that a plant containing large amounts of the fungus shouldn't be smoked. The weed advocates won an injunction, which nullified the rule. Kevin Jacoby, the lawyer leading the suit, admitted that the weed industry expects a new set of rules will be drawn up to set similar requirements. Jacoby noted that these new rules would likely take six to eight months to be instituted and that this years outdoor harvest is "not under threat."[6] He essentially said, "Yes, we see the writing on the wall and won't be able to sell products infected with the fungus much longer, but we can at least sell it and get paid this year!" The disregard for public health and local jurisdiction in the name of short-term profit mongering is appalling and in the open. The last big news on this front was published 8/30/23 ,in the Journal of Environmental Health Perspectives. Marijuana users, according to the article, had 22-27% more heavy metals in their blood than nonusers.[7] Apparently, selling toxic products is just part of doing business in the weed industry.

Not only is there a pushback by the weed industry on the legality of testing, in lots of specific ways the very idea of testing is in question. In their ideal world there wouldn't be any pesky health officials looking over the industry's shoulders to keep them from having heavy metals, carcinogens, and molds in their products; after all, that just gets in the way of profits.

Another line we were told that wouldn't be crossed, when Amendment 64 was proposed, is being jumped over and ignored regularly; the existence of consumption lounges. Although the idea rolls back decades of public health advancements that have made smoking indoors next to impossible, these spaces end up putting acutely intoxicated people out onto the streets and, of most concern, behind the wheel. The industry's argument against restricting these lounges was how unfair it was that people could drink in bars but not smoke weed in them. The moratorium on indoor consumption was first chipped away at with the introduction of mobile lounges, basically buses that people could use on. Since these buses didn't have a permanent address they drove through a loophole in the laws. But that wasn't nearly enough, the demand grew to allow for brick and mortar locations where people could use, mostly smoke, THC. For a little glimpse inside the mindset of these places, there is a video on google maps for "The Coffee Joint" in Denver. In the video, "Meredith" explains that "unfortunately because of our license we have to adhere to the Colorado indoor clean act," but you can come here and use edibles, dab rigs and vape flower. Now appearing are "articles that suggest that vaping flower gets you higher than smoking it".[8] In Colorado a law was passed called the "Colorado Marijuana Hospitality Establishment Act" (HB 19-1230). It created a legal exception to the Colorado Clean Air Act, allowing for onsite consumption.[9]

In my opinion, the biggest issue with these consumption sites is that, according to CDC as well as everyone who has ever been in a car where someone is smoking, second-hand smoke containing THC is intoxicating.[10] The difference between these places and the bars that they want to be like, is that I can go to a bar with friends as the "designated driver" and won't get drunk watching people drink. But the science suggests that nobody who spends more than a few minutes inside a closed room where THC is being smoked or vaped will escape intoxication. Since everyone leaving these places will be at some level intoxicated, no one should be driving afterwards. Right? The compromise I suggest is that they aren't allowed parking lots and everyone has to Uber home, but that's unlikely to gain much traction.

Another item on the hit list of the THC industry has been advertising. They are happy to agree to strict restrictions when it is up for a vote because they know all they have to do is later file suit, claiming that their first amendment right to free speech is being stepped on by those restrictions. The amount of kid-friendly advertisements for THC have been well documented over the years. I have heard directly from the mouths of THC lobbyists how they want to keep their products out of the hands of kids while fighting for expanded access and advertising. They want their wares marketed in public, but privately they know that the best customers are the ones who start early, use often, and like the strong stuff.

The "medical" label just keeps getting sillier and sillier. For example, Colorado added some interesting conditions under which a person can get their medical card. Originally the law allowed for "Severe Pain" which allowed pretty much anyone who wanted one to claim pain and get a card. Apparently that was too restrictive, so CO. voted to add PTSD.[11] The root of this problem is determining medicinal value by vote; removing the need to prove a product works. PTSD is a perfect example because the studies are so conflicting as to whether it helps PTSD or makes it worse. Multiple studies show it makes things worse, and a few that suggest it makes things better.[12] The problem arises when someone tells all of the good and none of the bad; remember the giant-less Jack and the beanstalk story? What people hear are stories about very sick people, typically children, that no one with an ounce of compassion would oppose giving relief to in any form. But the storyline quickly expands to include just about anybody, like me for example! While I was writing this I decided to test how silly it has gotten lately. I went online to get a card; that is possible in Colorado. In the past I would have had to talk to someone, but now it can be done completely online. In the process I was introduced to a company called, 'NuggMD.' Their homepage says it will only take minutes and you get a full refund if you don't get approved.[13] I now get regular emails from them encouraging me to finish applying, with descriptions of how lovely life will be with my Med Card. Medical marijuana has become an almost meaningless term.

Oklahoma "takes the cake" when it comes to lowering the criteria for access to medical marijuana. Their law says anyone can get a card if a physician signs off on it, and no one has to disclose what their condition is. Legally, any resident of that state over 21, can qualify. For those under the age of 21, they need a sponsor, who can get a med card and buy THC on their behalf.[14] As of this writing, there are over 2200 dispensaries in Oklahoma, making it the second highest concentration per capita in the country. I have visited a couple of times and the proliferation of weed is unlike anywhere else. Consult "Weedmaps" and look at the state. Since anyone can get a card they need LOTS of "Medical Retail." What started as a way to help relieve pain for very sick and dying patients and something to remove red tape for parents looking for CBD rich forms of cannabis to treat kids with seizure disorders, has become a joke. "Medical" has come to mean "as close to recreational as possible" and "recreational is coming soon."

The collective outrage that exists today towards big Pharma, like Purdue and the Sackler family, is well deserved but it was super late in coming. Apparently, Purdue convinced the world that any pain was a bad thing and needed to be medicated. THC is being sold in the same way.[15] The idea that we should avoid pain at any cost is new and it's not healthy. Pain is our body's way of telling us something is wrong and that we should deal with it, not just mask it. There are, of course, exceptions to this. In my life, not counting fingers and toes, I have broken 34 bones, including a neck that healed wrong, and 11 diagnosed concussions. One ER doctor, reviewing my chart, asked if I was a "rodeo rider or something"! (wish I were that tough.) Bottom line, I understand acute and chronic pain, I have plenty of days where that fog of pain is so thick I can't see through it but thankfully, I have chosen to deal with my pain in more productive ways than covering it with intoxication. I recommend the work of my dear friend Mel Pohl MD (A Day Without Pain and The Pain Antidote.) to those of you in similar situations.[16,17]

A recent article from a site called *solvingsudtogether.org* (SUD is Substance Use Disorder, aka addiction) describes a young man who details his struggle with prescription pain pills from a childhood snowboarding accident. He is now CEO of a weed shop and uses cannabis to control his cravings.[18] Substituting one high for another is dangerous ground, but there's a massive push to make this idea acceptable in the sober community.

Back to the original story, after the mouse gets his cookie and his glass of milk he wants a straw. Our industry mouse wants access to money and the mainstream financial system, proposed in "The Safe Banking Act" and "The Safer Banking Act".[19,20] At this point in time, weed shops cannot technically take credit cards, but they all do. They can't get traditional financing, they can't write off expenses (like advertisements), and most importantly, they can't take huge sums of cash into a bank and convert them into digital funds. One of the reasons America doesn't have bills larger than $100 is to make it hard for people making their money in illicit ways, drugs and human trafficking for example, to launder large sums of cash through established financial channels. As of this writing we are recklessly moving towards removing those restrictions and much of the money behind it all is, you guessed it, the weed industry.

In addition to everything else, they don't pay their taxes. That was the "silver lining" voters were told about and which helped garner support. Imagine, if you had an all cash (more or less) business, would you be walking down to your local IRS office all the time, making certain to pay them their share? There is a company in Oregon, called "American Patriot Brands," that owes the state $27m in back taxes![21] That's a small example of how corporate America hates paying taxes. They promise to pay but companies withhold and states misallocate. It's not new.

Have you heard of THC delivery services? Your kid sure has. Many states that allow recreational sales also allow home delivery. Young people love this because all that is required is someone to be there who is 21 to meet the driver; they can order whatever they want.

The advertisements are shocking, but the prize for the most outrageous has to go to a new chain called "The Dab." This brand was started by the company "Silverpeak," which started as a high-end store in downtown Aspen. The owner built this new brand focused, unapologetically, on concentrates. ("Dabbing" is a verb describing a type of concentrate consumption.) Their products cater to the low-end economic sector, to people looking for the most high for their dollar. Cruise their website, click the button verifying you are 21, and start shopping; includes delivery or in store pickup options. You will see on their site things like 1000mg's of live resin for $20 that comes in a syringe, and a pack of 100mg concentrate-infused gummys for $10. If you bring a friend in for the first time you're awarded 300 Loyalty Points. They advertise aggressively for the hardest users and then reward those users when they bring them new customers.[22]

The unscrupulous tactics these people will use are limitless. Recently I stumbled across a copy of the children's book, "It's Just a Plant," in the kids section at my local library.[23] It's safe to assume that if there is any way they can get away with something they will and if they can't they will pay to have the legal framework changed so they can.

According to the last "Monitoring the Future Survey", we know the current perception of risk associated with THC use has never been lower. Conversely, the negative effects of THC, because of the potency, have never been more severe.[24] We find ourselves in a situation where what people are using today is more damaging to their health but fewer people than ever believe there are any harms associated with it. My thesis is that we are now paying the price for overrepresentation of the harms of cannabis in years past. The sensationalistic fear tactics used in "Reefer Madness" and other materials like it, molded the nation's understanding of what was called, "the devil's lettuce." As a result, the ability to discuss the actual harms today has been compromised. Of great concern is how that gap is bridged, how do we begin to educate about risks associated with today's THC products when the general public has no confidence in any message that remotely sounds like "anti-weed"?

The problem probably has to get worse before it gets better. Between now and then, there is going to be a ton of collateral damage. There has already been so much suffering (don't forget "Johnny's Ambassadors"), that the thought of more is heartbreaking. Eleven years after Amendment 64 passed, there aren't many people left in my life who haven't been negatively impacted by the THC market in Colorado. Too many of my friends have sad stories, mostly of their kids, but also plenty of adults. Multiple friends relapsed inside of long-term recovery on THC; some made it back, some haven't, and some won't. My friends who have had kids experience psychosis, number in the double digits. I know several parents who lost their kids to their addiction, often to the ensuing psychosis after they started on concentrates. One of the disturbingly hopeful developments is how many white kids from wealthy families are showing up addicted to THC and experiencing severe mental illness as a result. There are even a couple of local politicians who have been affected personally and are talking about it. The sad reality is that it often takes this kind of needless suffering to move the needle. With that being said, the politics of this are tricky. Politicians are getting lots of donations from THC companies who are cash rich. Trulive financed almost the entire $40m for the ballot initiative in Florida this year. AS of this writing there has been less than $150 donated by anyone other than Trulive, that huge, Florida-based, multinational corporation.[25] The state's AG filed an injunction, saying the ballot language unfairly favors the company and "entrenches the sponsors monopolistic stranglehold on the marijuana market to the detriment of Floridians." For Trulive, dropping $40m into the campaign means they probably greasing the palms of local politicians all over the state.[26]

This was to be the end of the book, but a conversation with a friend, who runs a nonprofit in the addiction and recovery world, asked if psychedelics were addressed. My response was, "No, this is about THC, not other stuff." After a hard look, he said, "You wrote before how this thing is about all drugs, not just THC. We are watching phase three of the DPA (Drug Policy Alliance, a pro-weed advocacy group) plan which is 'medical psychedelics' so can we go back and explain what's next?" I didn't feel like writing anymore but kids are the ones who are paying the price. He was right, I shut up and started to write…

First, a caveat. Once more we're merrily skipping down the same road towards the same carnival and buying all of the nonsense the barker is yelling. We are turning something into medicine because we're hearing stories of individuals and seeing some interesting initial data. We are jumping over the safeguards that protect consumers and restrict corporations because there is huge money behind it all working to convince us that they should be allowed to sell whatever to whomever. I am talking about the marketing of psychedelics as medicine.

I work in addiction and mental health, it is my daily life. I also personally live with SUD and mental illness. Don't think for a second that I don't want to see new and improved treatments for people like me. Every tool we have can and should be deployed, but this particular "tool" isn't ready for prime time and it's already misunderstood by design.

There has been some compelling data for a while now about the use of small amounts of psychedelics to treat some intense conditions and improve some therapeutic outcomes.[27] It has been and continues to be seriously studied because there is likely efficacy in these treatments, that's why there continues to be real science and study going into the subject. I have a couple of friends who have personally participated in these studies. For one it was amazing, for the other nothing. With that said, these products are absolutely not ready for mainstream consumption and unregulated, unsupervised use. Another mood altering substance that can be taken until we feel what we want to feel is the last thing we need as a nation. Yet, it is the next thing the corporate drug dealers need to expand their businesses.

To sum up a bunch of relevant science, the idea of microdosing (a very small, measured and nonintoxicating amount of psychedelics), has real potential to help some people when used in some circumstances and managed by trained professionals. The problem is in the disparities between these two realities; people with SUD don't microdose anything, and those selling this need lots of people to use their products so they can make lots of money. So, the idea of microdosing appeals to every addict on earth because we know in our hearts we won't microdose for long. There's an old saying in the recovery world that for those of us with SUD, "if one is good, two is better." The very nature of addiction means we lose the ability to moderate or control our use. If we could control it we wouldn't be addicted! See the issue? Those who don't have SUD and compulsive tendencies will use small amounts, those of us with the bug will not be able to moderate that use. This is "understanding addiction 101;" it really can't get more straight forward. In the same way I don't push my experience on people as the only reality, others can't assume that their ability to moderate exists for everyone.

Not only has this plan been clearly stated in years past, more on that later, the results are so predictable and easy to see if one looks. Every weed-business-focused-publication I read is now talking about getting into psychedelic sales. The weed conferences all have workshops and lectures on getting into the business of selling these products and pushing for legislation allowing the sales. This is literally the same people who brought you corporate THC, who as evidenced prior, are in many cases literally the same people who brought us tobacco, alcohol and opiates. They are attempting to pull the same trick with different words. The time has come to tell them to stay out of our medicine cabinets and our wallets.

Recently I was sitting on a panel at a big conference of professional therapists alongside two amazing minds in the field that you met previously in the book; Latisha Bader and Christian Thurstone MD. One of the questioners asked if anyone else had sounded the alarm, other than myself. I laughed out loud because I was literally sitting between two of them. Dr. Thurstone had written white papers about what would happen and was sounding the alarm well before I was. I learned and continue to learn so much from his work. Dr. Bader was writing, speaking and teaching within a year of commercial sales happening and I could list dozens of others without an effort. Yes, there were MANY people sounding the alarm about the potential harms and unknowns of THC as well as the potency issues but mostly about allowing the industry to establish itself without proper oversight. When the salesmen see the money that can be made predicting their actions gets pretty easy.

In my first book, I shared the plan that the DPA shared with us and has since tried to cover up and whitewash. Here again is their strategy:

1. Medical Marijuana

2. Recreational Marijuana

3. Medical Psychedelics

4. Recreational Psychedelics

5. Medical Opiates (not directed by a doctor)

6. Recreational Opiates (pretty much happening in Canada)

7. Medical Stimulants (not the stuff we already have, cocaine and meth derivatives)

8. Recreational Stimulants

To again quote the Executive Director of the DPA when all of this was first happening in his TED talk "drugs are an undeveloped global commodity"[28]

The people behind these movements could care less about your physical and mental health, about the well-being of your family and your community. They care about your money and getting as much of it as they can. They have proven to us again and again that they will lie to get what they want and cheat to keep it. It is past time we stopped believing the people selling something to best represent that thing. It's time to turn our frustration and anger into action; it's time to, push back!

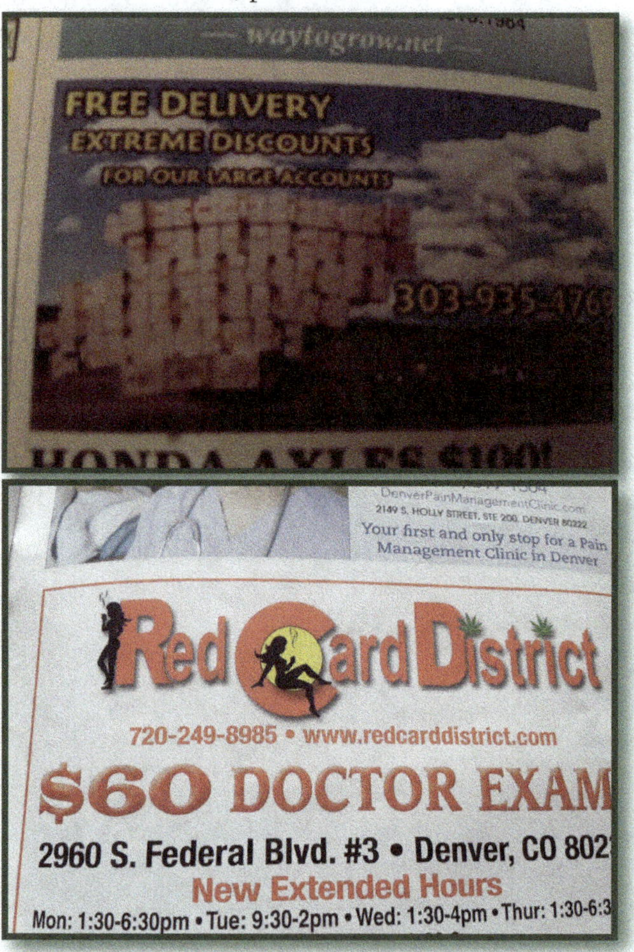

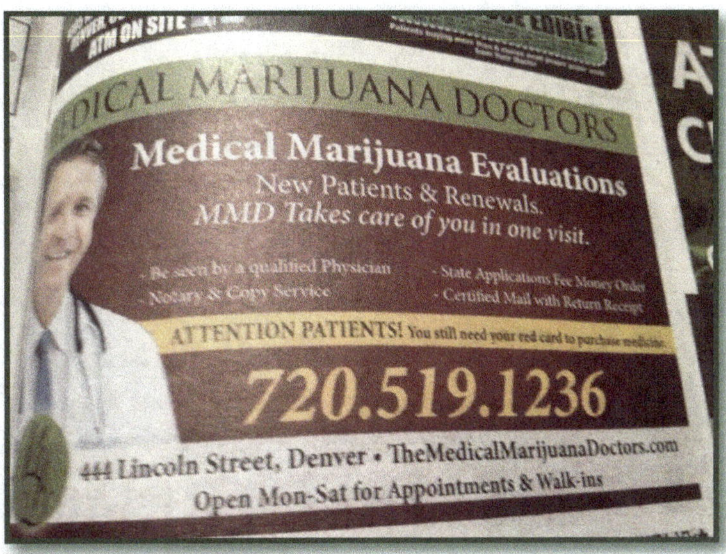
ATM ON SITE
EDIBLE
DICAL MARIJUANA DOCTORS
Medical Marijuana Evaluations
New Patients & Renewals.
MMD Takes care of you in one visit.
Be seen by a qualified Physician
Notary & Copy Service
State Applications Fee Money Order
Certified Mail with Return Receipt
ATTENTION PATIENTS! You still need your red card to purchase medicine.
720.519.1236
444 Lincoln Street, Denver • TheMedicalMarijuanaDoctors.com
Open Mon-Sat for Appointments & Walk-ins

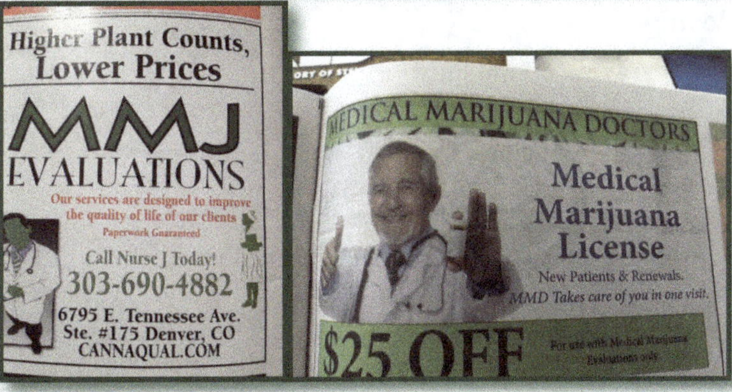
Higher Plant Counts,
Lower Prices
MMJ
EVALUATIONS
Our services are designed to improve
the quality of life of our clients
Paperwork Guaranteed
Call Nurse J Today!
303-690-4882
6795 E. Tennessee Ave.
Ste. #175 Denver, CO
CANNAQUAL.COM
MEDICAL MARIJUANA DOCTORS
Medical
Marijuana
License
New Patients & Renewals.
MMD Takes care of you in one visit.
$25 OFF
For use with Medical Marijuana
Evaluations only

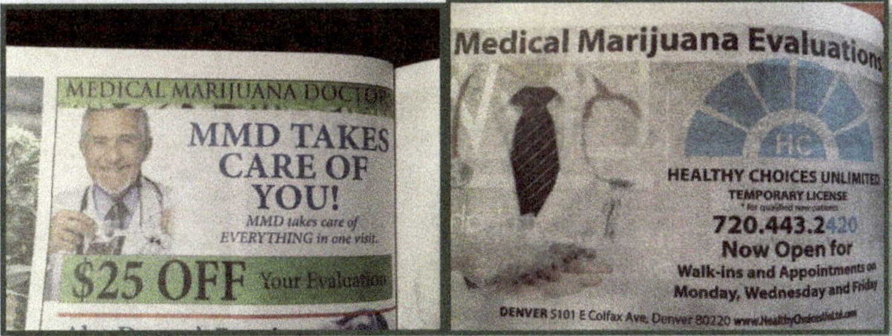
MEDICAL MARIJUANA DOCTOR
MMD TAKES
CARE OF
YOU!
MMD takes care of
EVERYTHING in one visit.
$25 OFF Your Evaluation
Medical Marijuana Evaluations
HEALTHY CHOICES UNLIMITED
TEMPORARY LICENSE
for qualified new patients
720.443.2420
Now Open for
Walk-ins and Appointments on
Monday, Wednesday and Friday
DENVER 5101 E Colfax Ave, Denver 80220 www.HealthyChoicesUnltd.com

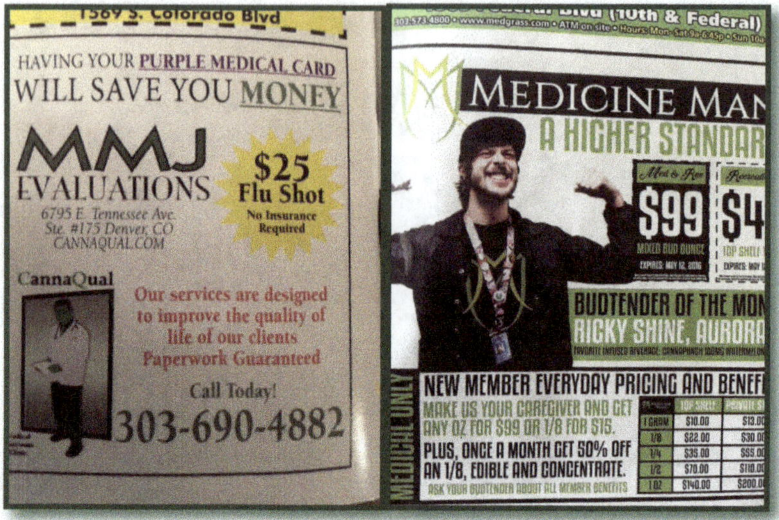

Closing

There isn't one community in the country that says, "What this town needs are more drugs." We have reached an unprecedented place in America. Overdose (OD) is the number one leading cause of accidental death. Our jails and prisons are full. The healthcare system is failing to treat SUD and many treating SUD have no idea what they are doing. We have drugs that can stop overdose that are now available over the counter, yet our OD numbers continue to rise. While opiates remain the leading cause of OD, amphetamines and alcohol are starting to catch up. We are trending in the wrong direction and the scary thing is that we are getting used to it in the same way that we got used to the idea of "super predators" and throwing away the key in the 90's. It took a while but society finally realized that throwing everyone in prison isn't working. How long will it take for us to come to the collective realization that letting people do whatever they want isn't working either. The ultra-liberalization of drug laws has been falsely tied to a desire to stop criminalizing addiction. As an addict who works all day with addicts I love aspects of this new awareness. Addicts aren't bad people but we often do things that hurt other people and ourselves in pursuit of our addiction. If left unchecked we will continue to do the same thing, we need help. We need help that gets to the root causes of addiction, not the typical "just say no" and to "pull yourselves up by your own bootstraps" mantras. We need medical care that includes long term psychiatric care and monitoring. We need to address the pain and trauma that drove most of us to use in the first place. We need to consider the hopeless futures that so many in America have because of where they are born and what resources they will have access to. If we want to actually address addiction and mental illness it is going to take a lot more than just not arresting addicts.

Now for the paradox; very few people just wake up and decide to get clean. That decision often comes because we face consequences for our use. I work with hundreds of addicts every year and almost no one asks for help because they have seen the light. We get help when we are in dire straits. The justice system is a good means to help us realize that we need help.

Oregon is the best example of what happens when groups like the DPA get their way, when the dog catches the car if you will. Sure, it's easy to say something isnt working but tricky to create something that actually works. In 2020 Oregon passed measure 110, making the possession of all drugs a fine, at worst.[29] The result has been a 53.3% increase in drug overdoses in the state compared to a 14% increase nationwide.[30,31] Oops! That one metric says all there is to say. They let the DPA literally write their dream law and more people died. They try to spin it in plenty of ways, like saying less people were arrested for drug use, but the reality is that this massive change in drug policy has been proven ineffective. As of this writing the data only considers 2021, but that shows a statewide increase in violent crimes increasing 11.8% in year one while the national average dropped 1.7%. Preliminary data for the first 6 months of 2022 shows a 3% increase on top of the year before.[32]

One of the solutions people, like the DPA, are starting to discuss seriously is that we have to regulate the drug supply, take it out of the black market, let corporate America fix this by selling drugs that will be "tightly regulated." This may sound good but I believe that by doing so we would ensure our place as the world's "highest" place and guarantee that the problem will grow as it becomes financially attractive to the salivating profiteers in suits and ties waiting to take over for the cartels.

Measure 110 did plenty to make stuff worse, but nothing compares with how it crippled drug court in the State. Drug courts work, there is ample evidence. Many argue that they are the single best tool we have to fight addiction and the data supports that.[33] In a nation that has screwed up its drug policy in almost every way imaginable, the drug courts stand out as a light of effectiveness. If you're not familiar I'll give you the broad brush explanation of how they work.

When a person gets arrested for something but the root cause of what they did is their addiction, the prosecutor and the defense attorney agree that this is a person who needs help for their addiction more than they need punishment for their crime so they offer them drug court. The deal is that the individual pleads guilty in exchange for a deferred sentence and then enters drug court. Drug court steps in with treatment when needed and support. They reward participants for productive behaviors and sanction them for destructive behaviors. By using the deferred sentence they can put a participant in jail for a day or two, or fine them, or take away something that they want when they use or don't follow the direction of the advocate. Most of these programs last about two years and have a tremendous success rate. At the end of the allotted time the participant "graduates" drug court and the original charge is dismissed.

When Oregon passed 104 they took away the ability to charge someone with a crime that would carry any real sentence, thereby removing the ability for the parties to agree to defer. Nobody is going to agree to enter an intensive program for two years to avoid a $100 fine, so nobody goes into drug court. Instead they languish in their addiction and become a statistic. The DPA claims that a person can't be forced to get clean, but neither can their addiction be ignored. Patrick Kennedy likes to say, "Meet people where they are, but don't leave them there." Policies like 110 leave people right where they are, addicted and hopeless.

I hope that you are beginning to see the complexities of drug policies. We don't want to go back to the insane sentences and criminalization of addiction of years past but neither do we want to remove effective tools to help those in need. We must move away from the silly all or nothing policies and oversimplification that seems to be ruling the day. This problem is very complex and the solution(s) will not fit on a bumper sticker. The legs of the stool are prevention, intervention and treatment. Making it even tougher, all three need to be quality. Unfortunately finding examples of any of these things done well is a challenge but that doesn't mean we stop trying! Is there anyone out there who wants to fund a think tank? For now, let me leave you with this; what we're doing isn't working. In the 12-step world we like to say, "Insanity is doing the same thing twice and expecting different results."

While earlier chapters have elaborated on my lack of faith in politicians to fix these issues, their hands can be forced and they will have to act if we demand it. Mental Healthcare in America today is in a sad state but it doesn't have to stay that way. We know how to prevent, how to intervene and how to treat; the knowledge is easy to access. I hope that we choose to apply what we know sooner than later because every day we delay not only can be but is someone's last.

If we continue to blindly buy all that the corporate powers that are BIG WEED are selling us, the responsibility will be on us as much as on them. We have seen this same story again and again in America, the rich get richer on the backs of the least fortunate. Anybody else feel like standing up and doing something about it this time?

NOTES AND REFERENCES

Chapter 1: Told ya so

1. Matt Zehner, "Brightfield's 2023 US Cannabis Market Forecast," *Brightfield Group,* February 21, 2023, https://blog.brightfieldgroup.com/brightfields-2023-us-cannabis-market-forecast#:~:text=What%20is%20the%20U.S.%20cannabis,to%20be%20worth%20%2450.7%20billion.

2. *Marihuana Tax Act* (1937)

3. United States Sentencing Commission, *Cocaine and Federal Sentencing Policy,* (United States Sentencing Commission, 1995), https://ussc.gov/sites/default/files/pdf/news/congressional-testimony-and-reports/drug-topics/199502-rtc-cocaine-sentencing-policy/1995-Crack-Report_Full.pdf.

4. "The American Alcohol Problem: An Overlooked and Deadly Epidemic," Blog, Caron, Last Accessed October 5, 2023, https://www.caron.org/blog/the-american-alcohol-problem.

5. Sonia Moghe, "Opioid history: From 'wonder drug' to abuse epidemic", *CNN health,* October 14, 2016, https://edition.cnn.com/2016/05/12/health/opioid-addiction-history/index.html.

6. "Tobacco-Related Mortality," CDC, Last Accessed September 28, 2023, https://www.cdc.gov/tobacco/data_statistics/fact_sheets/health_effects/tobacco_related_mortality/index.htm.

7. Saundra Young, "Marijuana stops child's severe seizures," *CNN health,* August 7, 2013, https://www.cnn.com/2013/08/07/health/charlotte-child-medical-marijuana.

8. "Colorado Revised Statutes 2016 CONSTITUTION OF THE STATE OF COLORADO," Leg.Colorado, 2016, https://leg.colorado.gov/sites/default/files/images/olls/crs2016-title-00.pdf.

9. "CBD, marijuana and hemp: What is the difference among these cannabis products, and which are legal?", *Michigan State University,* April 6, 2021, https://msutoday.msu.edu/news/2021/cbd-marijuana-and-hemp#:~:text=Hemp%20has%200.3%25%20or%20less,a%20compound%20found%20in%20cannabis.

10. Marc Crocq, "History of cannabis and the endocannabinoid system," *Dialogues in Clinical Neuroscience* 22, no. 3 (September 2020): 223-228, https://doi.org/10.31887/DCNS.2020.22.3/mcrocq.

11. Mahmoud ElSohly, et. al., "Changes in Cannabis Potency over the Last Two Decades (1995-2014) - Analysis of Current Data in the United States," *Biological Psychiatry* 79, no. 7 (April 2016): 613-619, https://doi.org/10.1016/j.biopsych.2016.01.004.

12. *The Agriculture Improvement Act* (2018)

13. Sinemyiz Atalay, Iwona Jarocka-Karpowicz, and Elzbieta Skrzydlewska, "Antioxidative and Anti-Inflammatory Properties of Cannabidiol," *Antioxidants* 9, no. 1 (January 2020): 21, https://doi.org/10.3390/antiox9010021.

14. Orrin Devinsky, et. al., "Cannabidiol: Pharmacology and potential therapeutic role in epilepsy and other neuropsychiatric disorders," *Epilepsia* 55, no. 6 (June 2014): 791-802, https://doi.org/10.1111/epi.12631.

15. Ákos Bajtel, et. al., "The Safety of Dronabinol and Nabilone: A Systematic Review and Meta-Analysis of Clinical Trials," *Pharmaceuticals* 15, no.1 (January 2022): 100, https://doi.org/10.3390/ph15010100.

16. F. Baratta, et. al., "Cannabis for Medical Use: Analysis of Recent Clinical Trials in View of Current Legislation," *Frontiers in Pharmacology* 13, (May 2022): 888903, https://doi.org/10.3389/fphar.2022.888903.

17. Leeds School of Business, *2020 Regulated Marijuana Market Update,* (Boulder, Leeds School of Business, 2020), https://sbg.colorado.gov/sites/sbg/files/2020-Regulated-Marijuana-Market-Update-Final.pdf.

18. "The Ultimate Guide to Cannabis Extract," *Precision Extraction Solutions,* Last Accessed October 1, 2023, https://precisionextraction.com/2021/04/cannabis-extract-guide/.

19. "7 Things You Need to Know about Cannabis Extracts," Canadian Centre on Substance Use and Addiction, Last Accessed September 14, 2023, https://www.ccsa.ca/sites/default/files/2019-07/CCSA-Things-You-Need-to-Know-about-Cannabis-Extracts-2019-en.pdf.

20. Cécile Henquet, et. al., "Prospective cohort study of cannabis use, predisposition for psychosis, and psychotic symptoms in young people," *BMJ* 330, (January 2005): 11, https://doi.org/10.1136/bmj.38267.664086.63.

21. "How Cannabis Wax is Made," *Media bros,* January 11, 2022, https://mediabros.store/blogs/news/how-cannabis-wax-is-made#:~:text=Generally%2C%20these%20marijuana%20concentrates%20are,oil%20(BHO)%20extraction%20process.

22. Max Sargent, "Shatter And Wax: What Are They And How Are They Made?", *Royal Queen Seeds,* February 16, 2022, https://www.royalqueenseeds.com/uk/blog-shatter-and-wax-what-are-they-and-how-are-they-made-n69.

23. "Making the Sauce: High Terpene Full Spectrum Extraction (HTFSE)," *Precision Extraction Solutions,* Last Accessed September 28, 2023, https://precisionextraction.com/2018/05/high-terpene-extraction-sauce/#:~:text=The%20Sauce%20is%20made%20with,cannabinoids%20contained%20within%20the%20plant.

24. "How is Live Resin Made", *Tribetokes,* Last Accessed September 28, 2023, https://tribetokes.com/how-is-live-resin-made.

25. Lo Friesen, "Solventless Extracts: An Overview," *cannabis science tech,* March 7, 2022, *https://www.cannabissciencetech.com/view/solventless-extracts-an-overview.*

26. "What is THC Distillate & How Do You Use It?", *LivWell,* Last Accessed September 28, 2023, https://livwell.com/blog/thc-distillate.

27. Priyamvada Sharma, Pratima Murthy, and Srinivas Bharath, "Chemistry, Metabolism, and Toxicology of Cannabis: Clinical Implications," *Iranian Journal of Psychiatry* 7, no.4 (2012): 149-156.

Chapter 2: The Rich Get Richer

1. Jeff Smith, "Seven US marijuana CEOs saw compensation top $4 million in 2021," *MJBizDaily,* last modified November 30, 2022, https://mjbizdaily.com/seven-us-marijuana-ceos-saw-compensation-top-4-million-in-2021/.

2. Rachel Aragon, "Georgia green lights two companies to grow medical cannabis," *Atlanta News First,* September 22, 2022, https://www.atlantanewsfirst.com/2022/09/22/georgia-green-lights-two-companies-grow-medical-cannabis/

3. "OMMU Update," Office of Medical Marijuana Use, September 8, 2023, https://knowthefactsmmj.com/wp-content/uploads/ommu_updates/2023/090823-OMMU-Update.pdf.

4. Chris Roberts, "Trulieve legal settlement comes amid scrutiny of racial bias in cannabis industry," *MJBizDaily,* April 27, 2023, https://mjbizdaily.com/trulieve-legal-settlement-comes-amid-scrutiny-of-racial-bias-in-cannabis-industry/.

5. Hazey Taughtme, "Trulieve Faces Backlash For Juneteenth Promotion," *Black Cannabis,* June 24, 2022, https://blackcannabismagazine.com/trulieve-faces-backlash-for-juneteenth-promotion/.

6. Graham Abbott, "Steve DeAngelo Calls for the Toppling of Corporate Cannabis," *Ganjapreneur,* September 30, 2023, https://www.ganjapreneur.com/steve-deangelo-op-ed-calls-for-the-return-of-small-cannabis-businesses/.

7. Steve DeAngelo Webpage – https://stevedeangelo.com/.

8. Steve DeAngelo (@stevedeangelo), "In the last five years we've seen many examples how NOT to legalize cannabis," Tweet, September 25, 2022, https://twitter.com/stevedeangelo/status/1566810102975279104.

9. "Topple the Pyramids" Topple the Pyramids, last accessed October 20, 2023, https://stevedeangelo.com/wp-content/uploads/2022/09/ToppleThePyramid.pdf.

10. "Meet 9 Of The Richest People In The Cannabis Industry", *Markets Insider*, December 3rd, 2021, https://markets.businessinsider.com/news/stocks/meet-the-10-richest-people-in-the-cannabis-industry-1031023434.

11. Jen Wieczner, "The marijuana billionaire who doesn't smoke weed," *Fortune*, January 16, 2019, https://fortune.com/longform/marijuana-weed-cannabis-tilray-stock/.

12. Nick O'Malley, "A hard sell in a dark market," *The Sydney Morning Herald*, April 24, 2010, https://www.smh.com.au/national/a-hard-sell-in-a-dark-market-20100423-tj3n.html

13. "About Tobacco Tactics," Tobacco Tactics, accessed October 4, 2023, https://tobaccotactics.org/.

14. Thomas Edward, "Is Big Tobacco Pivoting to Big Cannabis?," *High Times*, September 27th, 2022, https://hightimes.com/business/is-big-tobacco-pivoting-to-big-cannabis/#:~:text=One%20of%20the%20biggest%20tobacco,weed%20startup%20Sanity%20Group%20GmbH.&text=British%20American%20Tobacco%20announced%20Monday,marijuana%20startup%20Sanity%20Group%20GmbH.

15. "About Emblem," Emblem a Division of Aleafia Health, last accessed October 19, 2023, https://emblemcannabis.com/about.

16. Christopher Leonard, "How an Oil Theft Investigation Laid the Groundwork for the Koch Playbook," *Politico*, July 22, 2019, https://www.politico.com/magazine/story/2019/07/22/kochland-excerpt-senate-investigation-oil-theft-native-american-tribes-227412/

17. Mona Zhang, "Koch-backed group joins marijuana push after Zoom with Snoop Dogg," *Politico*, April 6, 2021, https://www.politico.com/news/2021/04/06/charles-koch-snoop-dogg-marijuana-legalization-479148.

18. "New State Markets Could Boost U.S. Legal Cannabis Sales to \$72B by 2030," *New Frontier*, March 21, 2022, https://newfrontierdata.com/cannabis-insights/new-state-markets-could-boost-u-s-legal-cannabis-sales-to-72b-by-2030/.

19. Rob Errera, "Eye-Popping Book and Reading Statistics [2023]," *Toner Buzz*, October 4, 2023, https://www.tonerbuzz.com/blog/book-and-reading-statistics/.

Chapter 3: The Potency Issue and Tolerance

1. Shalini Lynch, "Tolerance and Resistance to Drugs," *MSD Manual*, September 2022, https://www.msdmanuals.com/en-gb/home/drugs/factors-affecting-response-to-drugs/tolerance-and-resistance-to-drugs#:~:text=Tolerance%20is%20a%20person's%20diminished,drug%20usually%20effective%20against%20them.

2. Gwen Lapham, et. al., "Prevalence of Cannabis Use Disorder and Reasons for Use Among Adults in a US State Where Recreational Cannabis Use Is Legal," *Journal of the American Medical Association* 6, no.8 (August 2023), https://doi.org/10.1001/jamanetworkopen.2023.28934.

3. William Kerr and Yu Ye, "Estimating Usual Grams per Day of Marijuana Use from Purchases," *Addiction Research & Theory* 30, no.5 (March 2022): 360-367, https://doi.org/10.1080/16066359.2022.2049255.

4. "Regulating Marijuana Concentrates," Colorado General Assembly, last accessed October 2, 2023, https://leg.colorado.gov/bills/hb21-1317.

5. Mary Cash, et. al., "Mapping cannabis potency in medical and recreational programs in the United States," *PLOS One* 15, no.3 (March 2020), https://doi.org/10.1371/journal.pone.0230167.

6. Isabella Backman, "Not Your Grandmother's Marijuana: Rising THC Concentrations in Cannabis Can Pose Devastating Health Risks," *Yale School of Medicine,* August 30, 2023, https://medicine.yale.edu/news-article/not-your-grandmothers-marijuana-rising-thc-concentrations-in-cannabis-can-pose-devastating-health-risks/.

7. "Federal Food, Drug, and Cosmetic Act (FD&C Act)," FDA, March 29, 2018, https://www.fda.gov/regulatory-information/laws-enforced-fda/federal-food-drug-and-cosmetic-act-fdc-act.

8. "FDA History", FDA, June 29, 2018, https://www.fda.gov/about-fda/fda-history#:~:text=Although%20it%20was%20not%20known,and%20misbranded%20food%20and%20drugs.

9. Samuel Adams, *The Great American Fraud,* (Chicago: American Medical Association, 1905)

10. Cinnamon Bidwell, Renèe Willett, and Hollis Karoly, "Advancing the science on cannabis concentrates and behavioural health," *Drug and Alcohol Reviews* 40, no.6 (September 2021): 900-913, https://doi.org/10.1111/dar.13281.

11. Thomas Mitchell, "Colorado to Require Four-Page Warning With Marijuana Concentrate Sales," *Westword,* November 23, 2021, https://www.westword.com/marijuana/colorado-four-page-health-warning-marijuana-concentrate-sales-12763763.

12. "Use of Regulated Marijuana Concentrate," Colorado Department of Revenue Marijuana Enforcement Division, October 29, 2021, https://sbg.colorado.gov/sites/sbg/files/211101%20MED%20Educational%20Resource.pdf

Chapter 4: Black Market

1. *The Legalization Of Marijuana In Colorado: The Impact Volume 8* (Rocky Mountain HIDTA Investigative Support Center, 2021), https://www.rmhidta.org/_files/ugd/4a67c3_b391ac-360f974a8bbf868d2e3e25df3d.pdf

2. Christine Demont, Kylie Yocum, and Kirk Bol, "Drug Overdose Deaths in Colorado: Final Data for 2010-2020," *Health-*

Watch, January 2022, https://drive.google.com/file/d/1VGO-SUU15rxV-Zj37T5c9GW13w2D76uzm/view?pli=1.

3. "Drug Overdose Deaths," *Centers for Disease Control and Prevention,* last modified August 22, 2023, https://www.cdc.gov/drugoverdose/deaths/index.html.

4. "Arrest Offense Counts In The United States," Federal Bureau of Investigation, Crime Data Explorer, last accessed September 22, 2023, https://cde.ucr.cjis.gov/LATEST/webapp/#/pages/explorer/crime/arrest?link_id=3&can_id=35326d-6f88a15d5e75009aea804ac9a0&source=email-fbi-police-made-over-a-quarter-million-marijuana-arrests-in-2022&email_referrer=email_2083210&email_subject=fbi-police-made-over-a-quarter-million-marijuana-arrests-in-2022

5. "Marijuana Use Statistics Around the World (2019)," *Delphi Behavioral Health Group,* last accessed September 22, 2023, https://delphihealthgroup.com/marijuana/marijuana-global-use-statistics.

6. Beth Warren, "Cartel-backed pot grows linked to human trafficking inhumane working conditions," *USA Today,* June 18, 2023, https://www.usatoday.com/in-depth/news/nation/2023/06/18/cartel-backed-pot-grows-linked-to-california-oregon-human-trafficking/70329795007/#:~:text=Thousands%20of%20illegal%20marijuana%20grow,-public%20lands%20across%20Northern%20California.&text=TRINITY%20COUNTY%2C%20Calif.,-%E2%80%95%20Standing%20atop%20a.

7. "Cannabis Black Market Thrives Despite Legalization," *Rutgers Center of Alcohol and Substance Use Studies,* last accessed September 20, 2023, https://alcoholstudies.rutgers.edu/cannabis-black-market-thrives-despite-legalization/.

8. Lauren Weisner and Sharyn Adams, "A State and National Overview of Methamphetamine Trends," *ICJIA,* July 11, 2019, https://icjia.illinois.gov/researchhub/articles/illinois-and-national-methamphetamine-trends.

9. Vanda Felbab-Brown, *Fending off fentanyl and hunting down heroin* (Brookings Institution, 2020), https://www.brookings.edu/

wp-content/uploads/2020/07/9_Felbab-Brown_Mexico_final.pdf.

10. Roberto Secades-Villa et al., "Probability and predictors of the cannabis gateway effect: A national study," *International Journal of Drug Policy* 26, no.2 (February 2015): 135-142, https://doi.org/10.1016/j.drugpo.2014.07.011.

11. A.J. Herrington, "Gallup Poll Finds More Americans Smoke Marijuana Than Cigarettes," *Forbes,* August 29, 2022, https://www.forbes.com/sites/ajherrington/2022/08/29/gallup-poll-finds-more-americans-smoke-marijuana-than-cigarettes/?sh=4231d1d2b7a1.

12. Mike Bebernes, "Why hasn't legal weed killed the marijuana black market?," *Yahoo News,* December 16, 2022, https://news.yahoo.com/why-hasnt-legal-weed-killed-the-marijuana-black-market-224158722.html?guce_referrer=aHR0cHM6Ly93d3cuZ29vZ2xlLmNvbS8&guce_referrer_sig=AQAAABvkocckmIK-COWJDkqwbSTUOnzjlzpQ2dX5JHwDbk8guPqFkHdN_UWg6w6AMNiVAAMXfAlRwbSLHTxZnDhT9GfW2KXK-PRmtBNl-BkWG9geEcepQqIbVRWBr8lJA-iH5YH_YF0Vig-7eS_j3LfkrgfACaevAUD9Dvg5-Tnzq9Umbrz&guccounter=2.

13. Luis Chaparro, "The Sinaloa Cartel is losing its marijuana business, and El Chapo's sons are going after the 'premium weed' market to make up for it," *Insider,* December 13, 2022, https://www.businessinsider.com/sinaloa-cartel-aiming-to-corner-marijuana-market-in-mexico-2022-12?r=US&IR=T.

Chapter 5: Feds

1. Amelia Taylor, and Jason Birkett, "Pesticides in cannabis: A review of analytical and toxicological considerations," *Drug Testing and Analysis* 12, no.2 (February 2020): 180-190, https://doi.org/10.1002/dta.2747

2. Colorado Department of Revenue, Marijuana Enforcement Division, *2020 Regulated Marijuana Market Update*, December 23, 2021, 31, https://sbg.colorado.gov/sites/sbg/files/2020-Regulated-Marijuana-Market-Update-Final.pdf

3. "Colorado: 2020 Census," United States Census Bureau, August 25, 2021, https://www.census.gov/library/stories/state-by-state/colorado-population-change-between-census-decade.html

4. "Nicotine Products Tax," Colorado General Assembly, accessed October 4, 2023, https://leg.colorado.gov/agencies/legislative-council-staff/nicotine-products-tax#:~:text=The%20nicotine%20tax%20is%2030,on%20state%20revenue%20and%20spending.

5. "U.S. State Tobacco Taxes," Tobacco-Free Kids, last modified March 15, 2021, https://www.tobaccofreekids.org/what-we-do/us/state-tobacco-taxes

6. Colorado Constitution, amend. 64

7. "Lobbying Firm Profile: Forbes Tate Partners," Open Secrets, last modified October 24, 2023, https://www.opensecrets.org/federal-lobbying/firms/summary?cycle=2019&id=D000066687

Chapter 6: Workplace Safety and Driving

1. "Welcome to Labor Assistance Professionals," Labor Assistance Professionals, last accessed October 2, 2023, https://www.laborassistanceprofessionals.com/?zone=/unionactive/view_page.cfm&page=Welcome.

2. National Institute on Drug Abuse, *What are marijuana's effects,* (National Institutes of Health, 2020), https://nida.nih.gov/publications/research-reports/marijuana/what-are-marijuana-effects.

3. Sirichai Chayasirisobhon, "Mechanisms of Action and Pharmacokinetics of Cannabis," *The Permanente Journal* 25, no. 1 (March 2021): 19-200, https://doi.org/10.7812/TPP/19.200.

4. "Denver Marijuana DUI Defense Lawyer," Churchill DUI Defense, last accessed October 20, 2023, https://www.denverdui.com/marijuana-dui-attorney#:~:text=Blood%20Test%20in%20Marijuana%20DUIs&text=The%20legal%20limit%20has%20been,should%20reach%20a%20guilty%20verdict.

5. "Detect and Deter Workday Cannabis Use," Hound Labs, Last Accessed October 12, 2023, https://houndlabs.com/product-overview/.

6. Leirer Vo, Yesavage Ja, and Morrow Dg, "Marijuana carry-over effects on aircraft pilot performance," *Aviation, Space, and Environmental Medicine* 62, no. 3 (March 1991): 221-22.

7. "Pre-Employment Drug Testing Laws by State," *Paycor,* July 29, 2021, https://www.paycor.com/resource-center/articles/pre-employment-drug-testing-laws-by-state/.

Chapter 7: What Can't They Do

1. Katie Shapiro, "Infused everything: These cannabis products might surprise you," *The Cannabist,* June 28, 2016, https://www.thecannabist.co/2016/06/24/surprising-cannabis-infused-products/53443/.

2. "Edible dosing for beginners: with dosage chart by milligrams," *Leafly,* February 4, 2022, https://www.leafly.com/learn/consume/edibles/edible-dosing.

3. Douglas Roehler et al., "Cannabis-Involved Emergency Department Visits Among Persons Aged <25 Years Before and During the COVID-19 Pandemic — United States, 2019–2022," CDC *Morbidity and Mortality Weekly Report,* July 14, 2023, https://www.cdc.gov/mmwr/volumes/72/wr/mm7228a1.htm

4. Alex Halperin, "'You're not going to die': how to survive an edible marijuana overdose," *The Guardian,* November 19, 2018, https://www.theguardian.com/society/2018/nov/18/marijuana-cannabis-edibles-overdose-too-much.

Chapter 8: Mental Health

1. U.S. Department of Health and Human Services, *U.S Surgeon General's Advisory: Marijuana Use and the Developing Brain,* (Office of Surgeon General, 2019), https://www.hhs.gov/surgeongeneral/reports-and-publications/addiction-and-substance-misuse/advisory-on-marijuana-use-and-developing-brain/index.html.

2. Rajiv Radhakrishnan, Samuel Wilkinson, and Deepak Cyril D'Souza, "Gone to Pot – A Review of the Association between Cannabis and Psychosis," *Frontiers in Psychiatry* 5, (May 2014), https://doi.org/10.3389/fpsyt.2014.00054.

3. Martin-Santos R, et. al., "Acute effects of a single, oral dose of d9-tetrahydrocannabinol (THC) and cannabidiol (CBD) administration in healthy volunteers," *Current Pharmaceutical Design* 18, no.32 (2012): 4966-4979, https://doi.org/10.2174/138161212802884780.

4. Simon D. Spivack and Jan Vijg, "Study Suggests Why Most Smokers Don't Get Lung Cancer," *Einstein,* April 11, 2022, https://www.einsteinmed.edu/news/4756/study-suggests-why-most-smokers-dont-get-lung-cancer/.

5. Mara Di Forti, et.al., "The contribution of cannabis use to variation in the incidence of psychotic disorder across Europe (EU-GEI): a multicentre case-control study," *The Lancet* 6, no.5 (May 2019): 427-436, https://doi.org/10.1016/S2215-0366(19)30048-3.

6. "Colorado Suicide Statistics," Colorado Department of Public health and Environment, last accessed October 23, 2023, https://cdphe.colorado.gov/colorado-suicide-statistics.

7. Beth Han, et.al., "Associations of Suicidality Trends with Cannabis Use as a Function of Sex and Depression Status," *Journal of the American Medical Association* 4, no. 6 (June 2021), https://doi.org/10.1001/jamanetworkopen.2021.13025.

8. Edmund Silins, et. al., "Young adult sequelae of adolescent cannabis use: an integrative analysis," *The Lancet* 1, no.4 (September 2014): 286-93, https://doi.org/10.1016/S2215-0366(14)70307-4.

9. "Marijuana," *History,* October 10, 2019, https://www.history.com/topics/crime/history-of-marijuana.

Chapter 9: 'Merica!

1. "Religion affiliation in Uruguay as of 2020 by type," Statista, October 17, 2023, https://www.statista.com/statistics/1067190/uruguay-religion-affiliation-share-type/.

2. Andres Figueras Arioso, "Legal marijuana, but Uruguayans still prefer black market," *Medical Press*, September 30, 2022, https://medicalxpress.com/news/2022-09-legal-marijuana-uruguayans-black.html.

3. Deon Mass, "Cannabis Compliance In Uruguay – Background Info, Fees & How-To Checklist [Free Licensing Guide]," *Cannavigia*, May 4, 2022, https://cannavigia.com/cannabis-country-report-uruguay-how-to-legally-grow-and-obtain-cannabis#:~:text=Only%20two%20strains%20of%20cannabis%20with%20a%20maximum,average%20monthly%20purchase%20was%207.8%20grams%2Fmonth%20per%20buyer.

4. "Cannabis Policy in The Netherlands: Moving Forwards Not Backwards." *Transform Drug Policy Foundation*, November 16, 2018, https://transformdrugs.org/blog/cannabis-policy-in-the-netherlands-moving-forwards-not-backwards#:~:text=Another%20widely%20reported%20move%20was,commensurate%20with%20its%20legal%20status.

5. Antoinette Radford, "Amsterdam bans cannabis in its red light district," *BBC News*, February 9, https://www.bbc.com/news/world-europe-64591394.

6. Mick Krever and Amararchi Orie, "Amsterdam is banning marijuana use on streets of red light district," *CNN Travel*, February 10, 2023, https://edition.cnn.com/travel/article/amsterdam-ban-marijuana-red-light-district-intl-scli/index.html#:~:text=Sidewalks%20are%20often%20packed%20with,Red%20Light%20district%20in%20Amsterdam.&text=In%20a%20bid%20to%20improve,city's%20legal%20sex%20work%20trade.

7. Mother Jones and Alex Park, "10 Supreme Court Rulings That Turned Corporations Into People," *AlterNet*, July 10, 2014, https://www.alternet.org/2014/07/10-supreme-court-rulings-turned-corporations-people.

8. Stephen Lim, et. al., "Measuring human capital: a systematic analysis of 195 countries and territories, 1990–2016," *The Lancet* 392, no.10154 (October 2018): 1217-1234, https://doi.org/10.1016/S0140-6736(18)31941-X.

9. Doug Fine, *Too High to Fail,* (New York: Penguin Group, 2013)

Chapter 10: Environment

1. Luke Sumpter, "How To Water Cannabis Plants: A Comprehensive Guide," Royal Queen Seeds, last modified December 28, 2022, https://www.royalqueenseeds.com/blog-how-to-water-cannabis-plants-a-comprehensive-guide-n1205

2. Michael Derewenko, "Water Demands for Cannabis," Jain by Rivulis, last modified June 20, 2021, https://jainsusa.com/blog/water-demands-for-cannabis/

3. Laura Drotleff, "Cannabis Requires More Water than Commodity Crops, Researchers Say," *MJBizDaily*, November 10, 2021, https://mjbizdaily.com/cannabis-requires-more-water-than-commodity-crops-researchers-say/

4. Zhonghua Zheng, Kelsey Fiddes & Liangcheng Yang, "A Narrative Review on Environmental Impacts of Cannabis Cultivation," *Journal of Cannabis Research* 3, no.35 (April 2021), https://doi.org/10.1186/s42238-021-00090-0

5. Colorado Department of Revenue, Marijuana Enforcement Division, *2020 Regulated Marijuana Market Update*, December 23, 2021, 31, https://sbg.colorado.gov/sites/sbg/files/2020-Regulated-Marijuana-Market-Update-Final.pdf

6. Colorado Department of Revenue, Marijuana Enforcement Division, *MED 2020 Annual Update*, September 17, 2021, 3, https://sbg.colorado.gov/sites/sbg/files/210916%202020%20MED%20Annual%20Final.pdf

7. "About: Mammoth Farms," Mammoth Farms, accessed April 7, 2023, https://www.mammothfarms.com/about

8. Brian Sparks, "North America's Largest Cannabis Growers for 2021," *Greenhouse Grower*, January 22, 2021, https://www.

greenhousegrower.com/crops/north-americas-largest-canna-bis-growers-for-2021/

9. Richard Heim and Richard Tinker, "National Drought Summary for September 26, 2023," U.S. Drought Monitor, September 28, 2023, https://droughtmonitor.unl.edu/Summary.aspx

10. Mike Noren, "How Much Water Does The Average Person Use Per Month?" Save the Drop LA, accessed April 7, 2023, https://savethedropla.com/how-much-water-does-the-average-person-use-per-month/

11. Beau Whitney and Beau Wilberding, *2022 U.S. Cannabis Supply Report* (Portland: Whitney Economics LLC, 2022).

12. Paige St. John, "The Reality of Legal Weed In California: Huge Illegal Grows, Violence, Worker Exploitation And Deaths," *Los Angeles Times*, September 8, 2022, https://www.latimes.com/california/story/2022-09-08/reality-of-legal-weed-in-califor-nia-illegal-grows-deaths

13. Iman Saleh et al., "Removal of pesticides from water and waste-water: Chemical, physical and biological treatment approaches," *Environmental Innovation and Technology* 19, (August 2020), https://doi.org/10.1016/j.eti.2020.101026

14. Evan Mills, "The Carbon Footprint of Indoor Cannabis Pro-duction," *Energy Policy* 46, (July 2012): 58-67, https://doi.org/10.1016/j.enpol.2012.03.023

15. Hailey M. Summers, Evan Sproul, and Jason C. Quinn, "The Greenhouse Gas Emissions of Indoor Cannabis Production in The United States," *Nature Sustainability* 4, (July 2021): 644-650, https://doi.org/10.1038/s41893-021-00691-w

16. "Short-Term Energy Outlook," U.S. Energy Information Ad-ministration, last modified October 11, 2023, https://www.eia.gov/outlooks/steo/report/electricity.php

Chapter 11: Medicine and Science and Shit

1. Bausch Health Companies Inc., Cesamet (nabilone) [prescribing information], U.S. Food and Drug Administration, last modi-

fied April 28, 2022, https://www.accessdata.fda.gov/drugsatf-da_docs/label/2022/018677Orig1s017lbl.pdf

2. GW Pharmaceuticals, Epidiolex (cannabidiol) [prescribing information], U.S. Food and Drug Administration, last modified October 20, 2023, https://www.accessdata.fda.gov/drugsatf-da_docs/label/2023/210365s020lbl.pdf

3. Alkem Laboratories, Marinol (dronabinol) [prescribing information], U.S. Food and Drug Administration, last modified January 17, 2023, https://www.accessdata.fda.gov/drugsatfda_docs/label/2023/018651s033lbl.pdf

4. GW Pharmaceuticals, Sativex [prescribing information], Jazz Pharmaceuticals Canada, last modified December 11, 2019, https://pp.jazzpharma.com/pi/sativex.ca.PIL-en.pdf

5. GW Pharmaceuticals, Epidiolex (cannabidiol) [prescribing information], U.S. Food and Drug Administration, last modified October 20, 2023, https://www.accessdata.fda.gov/drugsatf-da_docs/label/2023/210365s020lbl.pdf

6. Laura E. Ewing et al., "Hepatotoxicity of a Cannabidiol-Rich Cannabis Extract in the Mouse Model," *Molecules* 24, no. 9 (April 2019): 1694, https://doi.org/10.3390/molecules24091694

7. "Cannabidiol Drug Interactions," Drugs.com, last modified October 1, 2023, https://www.drugs.com/drug-interactions/can-nabidiol-index.html

8. Marcel O. Bonn-Miller et al., "Labeling Accuracy of Cannabidiol Extracts Sold Online," *Journal of the American Medical Association* 318, no.17 (November 2017): 1708-1709, bttps://doi.org/10.1001/jama.2017.11909

9. Hannah Gardener, Chela Wallin, and Jaclyn Bowen, "Heavy Metal and Phthalate Contamination and Labeling Integrity in a Large Sample of US Commercially Available Cannabidiol (CBD) Products," *The Science of the Total Environment* 851, no.1 (December 2022), https://doi.org/10.1016/j.scitotenv.2022.158110

10. Bill Gurley et al., "Content versus Label Claims in Cannabidiol (CBD)-Containing Products Obtained from Commercial Outlets in the State of Mississippi," *Journal of Dietary Supplements* 17,

no.5 (May 2020): 599–607, https://doi.org/10.1080/19390211.2020.1766634

11. Acabada Active Wear Website – https://acabadaactive.com/

12. NUFABRX 'Pain Relieving Apparel' Website – https://nufabrx.com/

13. Timothy Legg, "Is the Placebo Effect Real?" *Medical News Today*, September 7, 2017, https://www.medicalnewstoday.com/articles/306437#clinical-usage-of-placebos

14. Samuel T. Wilkinson, Elina Stefanovics, and Robert A. Rosenheck, "Marijuana Use is Associated with Worse Outcomes in Symptom Severity and Violent Behavior in Patients with Posttraumatic Stress Disorder," *The Journal of Clinical Psychiatry* 76, no.9 (September 2015): 1174-1180, https://doi.org/10.4088/JCP.14m09475

15. "Drug Scheduling," United States Drug Enforcement Administration, accessed October 4, 2023, https://www.dea.gov/drug-information/drug-scheduling#:~:text=Schedule%20I%20drugs%2C%20substances%2C%20or,)%2C%20methaqualone%2C%20and%20peyote

Chapter 12: All the nonsense or "Thank you 2018 farm bill"

1. "Farm Bill", U.S. Department of Agriculture, December 20, 2018, https://www.usda.gov/farmbill.

2. "THCA and THC: What's the difference?", *Weedmaps*, June 20, 2022, https://weedmaps.com/learn/cannabis-and-your-body/difference-between-thca-thc.

3. Dario Sabaghi, "What Is THC-O Acetate, And Why Is It Getting Attention?", *Forbes*, January 18, 2022, https://www.forbes.com/sites/dariosabaghi/2022/01/18/what-is-thc-o-acetate-and-why-is-it-getting-attention/?sh=2965d2f35991.

4. "Tetrahydrocannabinol acetate," PubChem, last accessed September 28, 2023, https://pubchem.ncbi.nlm.nih.gov/compound/Tetrahydrocannabinol-acetate#section=Related-Compounds.

5. Shanti Ryle, "What Is THCP?", *Leaf Well,* Last Accessed October 26, 2023, https://leafwell.com/blog/what-is-thcp.

6. Jeffrey Chen, "Unpacking the Hype Around THCV, aka 'Diet Weed'," *healthline,* August 19, 2021, https://www.healthline.com/health/substance-use/thcv.

7. Max Levenson, "What is HHC?", *Leafly,* August 24, 2022, https://www.leafly.com/news/strains-products/what-is-hhc.

8. "How Is HHC Totally Different From THC Or Delta-8?", *Buy HHC UK and Ireland,* May 29, 2022, https://buyhhcukandireland.com/hhc-news/how-is-hhc-totally-different-from-thc-or-delta-8/#:~:text=Ray%20delineated%20HHC%20producing%20as,that%20stage%E2%80%9D%20before%20distilling%20it.

9. "5 Things to Know about Delta-8 Tetrahydrocannabinol – Delta-8 THC", FDA, May 4, 2022, https://www.fda.gov/consumers/consumer-updates/5-things-know-about-delta-8-tetrahydrocannabinol-delta-8-thc.

Chapter 13: Kids/Parents

** no references needed but added section here in case you wanted to add a note

Chapter 14: To the Provider

1. Kenneth Finn, *Cannabis in Medicine: An Evidence-Based Approach* (Colorado Springs: Springer, 2020).

2. American Psychiatric Association, "Substance-Related and Addictive Disorders," in *Diagnostic and Statistical Manual of Mental Disorders*, Fifth Edition (Arlington, VA: American Psychiatric Association, 2013), 517–518.

Chapter 15: To the User

1. Divya Ramesh, Joel E. Schlosburg, Jason M. Wiebelhaus, and Aron H. Lichtman, "Marijuana Dependence: Not Just Smoke and Mirrors," *ILAR Journal* 52, no.3 (January 2011): 295-308, https://doi.10.1093/ilar.52.3.295

2. American Psychiatric Association, "Substance-Related and Addictive Disorders," in *Diagnostic and Statistical Manual of Mental Disorders*, Fifth Edition (Arlington, VA: American Psychiatric Association, 2013), 517–518.

Chapter 16: Women and Weed

1. Piazza NJ, Peterson JS, Yates JW, & Sundgren AS (1986). Progression of symptoms in women alcoholics: Comparison of Jellinek's model with two groups. Psychological Reports, 59, 367–370. [PubMed: 3786612]

2. Piazza NJ, Vrbka JL, & Yeager RD (1989). Telescoping of alcoholism in women alcoholics. The International Journal of the Addictions, 24(1), 19–28. [PubMed: 2759762]

3. Substance Abuse and Mental Health Services Administration (2009) National Survey on Drug Use and Health. MD: SAMHSA Center.

4. Becker JB, McClellan ML, and Glover Reed B (2017). Sex Differences, Gender and Addiction. Department of Psychology and the Molecular and Behavioral Neuroscience Institute, University of Michigan, Ann Arbor, MI 48109.

5. National Institutes of Health (NIH). *Amendment: NIH Policy and Guidelines on the Inclusion of Women and Minorities as Subjects in Clinical Research.*; 2001. https://grants.nih.gov/grants/guide/notice-files/NOT-OD-02-001.html.

6. Clayton JA, Collins FS. (2014) Policy: NIH to balance sex in cell and animal studies. *Nature.* 2014;509 (7500):282-283.

7. NIDA. 2021, April 13. The Importance of Including Women in Research . Retrieved from https://nida.nih.gov/publications/research-reports/substance-use-in-women/importance-including-women-in-research

8. National Bioethics Advisory Commission -- Publications. https://bioethicsarchive.georgetown.edu/nbac/pubs.html. Published 2001. Accessed January 24, 2018.

9. Treatment Improvement Protocol (TIP) Series, No. 51. HHS Publication No. (SMA) 13-4426.

10. NIDA. 2020, January 22. Substance Use in Women Drug Facts. Retrieved from https://nida.nih.gov/publications/drugfacts/substance-use-in-women on 2023, November 3

11. Substance Abuse and Mental Health Services Administration (2022) National Survey on Drug Use and Health. MD: SAMHSA Center.

12. Blanton HL, Barnes RC, McHann MC, Bilbrey JA, Wilkerson JL, Guindon J. (2021). Sex differences and the endocannabinoid system in pain. Pharmacol Biochem Behav. Mar;202:173107. doi: 10.1016/j.pbb.2021.173107. Epub 2021 Jan 12. PMID: 33444598; PMCID: PMC8216879.

13. American Psychiatric Association. (2013). *Diagnostic and statistical manual of mental disorders* (5th ed.). https://doi.org/10.1176/appi.books.9780890425596

14. Herrmann ES, Weerts EM, Vandrey R. (2015) Sex differences in cannabis withdrawal symptoms among treatment-seeking cannabis users. Exp Clin Psychopharmacol. 2015 Dec;23(6):415-21. doi: 10.1037/pha0000053. Epub 2015 Oct 12. PMID: 26461168; PMCID: PMC4747417.

15. Substance Abuse and Mental Health Services Administration (2018) National Survey on Drug Use and Health. MD: SAMHSA Center.

16. Dickson B, Mansfield C, Guiahi M, Allshouse AA, Borgelt LM, Sheeder J, Silver RM, Metz TD. (2018) Recommendations from cannabis dispensaries about first-trimester cannabis use. Obstet Gynecol. 2018;131:1031–38.

17. Gunn JKL, Rosales CB, Center, CB, Center KE, Nunez A, Gibson SJ, Christ, C and Ehiri. (2015) Prenatal exposure to cannabis and maternal and child health outcomes: a systematic review and meta-analysis British Journal of Medicine.

18. Substance Abuse and Mental Health Services Administration (2019) National Survey on Drug Use and Health. MD: SAMHSA Center.

19. Lynn BK, López JD, and Miller C (2019). The Relationship between Marijuana Use Prior to Sex and Sexual Function in Women. Sex Med;7:192–197.

20. Brazill, W (2021). Why Mommy Gets High: A Conversation Starter for Parents Who Get High.

21. Ilnitsky S and Van Uum S (2019) Marijuana and fertility. *CMAJ* 2019 June 10;191:E638. doi: 10.1503/cmaj.181577 *CMAJ* Podcasts: author interview at https://soundcloud.com/cmajpodcasts/181577-five

22. Leung J, Chan GCK, Hides L, Hall WD. (2020) What is the prevalence and risk of cannabis use disorders among people who use cannabis? a systematic review and meta-analysis. Addict Behav. 2020 Oct;109:106479. doi: 10.1016/j.addbeh.2020.106479. Epub 2020 May 20. PMID: 32485547.

23. MacKenzie, A., and Cservenka, A. (2023). Cannabis and emotion processing: A review of behavioral, physiological, and neural responses. *Experimental and Clinical Psychopharmacology, 31*(1), 263–279. https://doi.org/10.1037/pha0000529

24. Barbosa-Leiker C, Brooks O, Smith CL, Burduli E, Gartstein MA. Healthcare professionals' and budtenders' perceptions of perinatal cannabis use. Am J Drug Alcohol Abuse. 2022 Mar 4;48(2):186-194. doi: 10.1080/00952990.2021.1988091. Epub 2021 Nov 15. PMID: 34779673; PMCID: PMC9107527.

25. Peiper NC, Gourdet C, Meinhofer A, Reiman A, Reggente N. (2017) Medical decision-making processes and online behaviors among cannabis dispensary staff. Subst Abuse. 2017;11:1178221817725515.

26. Haug NA, C D, Sottile JE, Babson KA, Vandrey R, Bonn-Miller MO. Training and practices of cannabis dispensary staff. Cannabis Cannabinoid Res. 2016;1:244–51. doi:https://doi.

org/10.1089/can.2016.0024. [Crossref], [PubMed], [Google Scholar]

27. Forray A, Merry B, Lin H, Ruger JP, Yonkers KA. (2015) Perinatal substance use: a prospective evaluation of abstinence and relapse. Drug Alcohol Depend. 2015 May 1;150:147-55. doi: 10.1016/j.drugalcdep.2015.02.027. Epub 2015 Mar 3.: 25772437; PMCID: PMC4387084.

28. Gunn JKL, Rosales CB, Center KE, Nuñez A, Gibson SJ, Christ C, Ehiri JE (2016). Prenatal exposure to cannabis and maternal and child health outcomes: a systematic review and meta-analysis. *BMJ Open* 2016;**6:**e009986. doi: 10.1136/bmjopen-2015-009986

29. Brown QL, Sarvet AL, Shmulewitz D, Martins SS, Wall MM, Hasin DS. (2017) Trends in marijuana use among pregnant and nonpregnant reproductive-aged women, 2002-2014. Jama. 317:207–09.

30. Volkow ND, Han B, Compton WM, McCance-Katz EF. (2019). Self-reported medical and nonmedical cannabis use among pregnant women in the United States. JAMA;322:167.

31. Bailey BA, Wood DL, Shah D. (2020) Impact of pregnancy marijuana use on birth outcomes: results from two matched population-based cohorts. J Perinatol. 2020 Oct;40(10):1477-1482. doi: 10.1038/s41372-020-0643-z. Epub 2020 Mar 5. PMID: 32139807.

32. Ko JY, Farr SL, Tong VT, Creanga AA, Callaghan WM. (2015) Prevalence and patterns of marijuana use among pregnant and nonpregnant women of reproductive age. Am J Obstet Gynecol 2015;213:201.e1–10.

33. Ko JY, Coy KC, Haight SC, Haegerich TM, Williams L, Cox S, Njai R, Grant AM (2017). Characteristics of Marijuana Use During Pregnancy - Eight States, Pregnancy Risk Assessment Monitoring System. MMWR Morb Mortal Wkly Rep. 2020 Aug 14;69(32):1058-1063. doi: 10.15585/mmwr.mm6932a2. PMID: 32790656; PMCID: PMC7440118.

34. Besse M, Parikh K, Mark K. (2023) Reported Reasons for Cannabis Use Before and After Pregnancy Recognition. J Addict Med. 2023 Sep-Oct 01;17(5):563-567. doi: 10.1097/ADM.0000000000001178. Epub 2023 May 17. PMID: 37788610.

35. Rompala G, Nomura Y, Hurd YL. (2021). Maternal cannabis use is associated with suppression of immune gene networks in placenta and increased anxiety phenotypes in offspring. Proc Natl Acad Sci U S A. 2021 Nov 23;118(47):e2106115118. doi: 10.1073/pnas.2106115118. PMID: 34782458; PMCID: PMC8617511.

36. Drugs and Lactation Database (LactMed®) [Internet]. Bethesda (MD): National Institute of Child Health and Human Development; 2006-. Available from: https://www.ncbi.nlm.nih.gov/books/NBK501922/

37. Dodge P, Nadolski K, Kopakau H, Zablocki V, Forrestal K, Bailey B (2023) The impact of timing in utero marijuana exposure on fetal growth. Frontier Pediatrics, 16 May 2023. Sec Children and Health; Vol 11. https://doi.org/10.3389/fped.2023.1103749

38. Jones HE, Fielder A. (2015) Neonatal abstinence syndrome: Historical perspective, current focus, future directions. *Prev Med.* 2015;80:12-17. doi:10.1016/j.ypmed.2015.07.017

39. 39. Pan IJ, Yi HY. (2013). Prevalence of hospitalized live births affected by alcohol and drugs and parturient women diagnosed with substance abuse at liveborn delivery: United States, 1999-2008. Matern Child Health J;17:667–76.

40. National Institutes of Health (2013) Tobacco, drug use in pregnancy can double risk of stillbirth. https://www.nichd.nih.gov/newsroom/releases/121113-stillbirth-drug-use

41. Renard J & Konefal S (2020). Clearing the Smoke on Cannabis: Cannabis Use During Pregnancy and Breastfeeding – an update. Canadian Centre on Substance Use and Addiction.

42. Drugs and Lactation Database (LactMed®) [Internet]. Bethesda (MD): National Institute of Child Health and Human Development; 2006-. Cannabis. [Updated 2023 Apr 15].

43. Davis E, Lee T, Weber JT, Bugden S. (2020). Cannabis use in pregnancy and breastfeeding: The pharmacist's role. Can Pharm J (Ott). 2020 Jan 8;153(2):95-100. doi: 10.1177/1715163519893395. PMID: 32206154; PMCID: PMC7079319.

44. Wymore EM, Palmer C, Wang GS, Metz TD, Bourne DWA, Sempio C, Bunik M (2021). Persistence of Δ-9-Tetrahydrocannabinol in Human Breast Milk. JAMA Pediatr. 2021 Jun 1;175(6):632-634. doi: 10.1001/jamapediatrics.2020.6098. PMID: 33683306; PMCID: PMC7941249.

45. Joyce KM, Thompson K, Good KP (2021). The impact of depressed mood and coping motives on cannabis use quantity across the menstrual cycle in those with and without pre-menstrual dysphoric disorder. *Addiction*. Published online March 2, 2021.

46. Garner CD, Kendall-Tackett K, Young C, Baker T, Hale TW. (2022). Mode of Cannabis Use and Factors Related to Frequency of Cannabis Use Among Breastfeeding Mothers: Results from an Online Survey. Breastfeed Med. 2022 Mar;17(3):269-276. doi: 10.1089/bfm.2021.0151. Epub 2021 Dec 3. PMID: 34870449.

47. Miller AP, Baranger DAA, Paul SE, Hatoum AS, Rogers C, Bogdan R, Agrawal A. (2023) Characteristics Associated With Cannabis Use Initiation by Late Childhood and Early Adolescence in the Adolescent Brain Cognitive Development (ABCD) Study. JAMA Pediatr. 2023 Jun 26. doi: 10.1001/jamapediatrics.2023.1801. Epub ahead of print. PMID: 37358866

48. Reece AS and Hulse GK (2021). A geospatiotemporal and causal inference epidemiological exploration of substance and cannabinoid exposure as drivers of rising US pediatric cancer rates. *BMC Cancer* **21,** 197 (2021).

49. Reece AS and Hulse GK (2021). Cannabinoid exposure as a major driver of pediatric acute lymphoid Leukemia rates across the USA: combined geospatial, multiple imputation and causal inference study. *BMC Cancer* **21,** 984 (2021).

50. Graves LE, Robert M, Allen, VM, Dama S, Gabrys RL, Tanguay RL, Turner SD, Green CR, Cook JL (2022). Guideline No. 425b: Cannabis Use Throughout Women's Lifespans — Part 2: Pregnancy, the Postnatal Period, and Breastfeeding. Journal of Obstetrics and Gynaecology Canada, Volume 44, Issue 4, 2022, Pages 436-444.e1, ISSN 1701-2163, https://doi.org/10.1016/j.jogc.2022.01.013.

51. American College of Obstetricians and Gynecologists (October 2017) Marijuana Use During Pregnancy and Lactation. ACOG Committee Opinion. Number 722.

52. Joyce KM, Thompson K, Good KP, Tibbo PG, O'Leary ME, Perrot TS, Hudson A, Stewart SH. (2021) The impact of depressed mood and coping motives on cannabis use quantity across the menstrual cycle in those with and without pre-menstrual dysphoric disorder. Addiction. 2021 Oct;116(10):2746-2758. doi: 10.1111/add.15465. Epub 2021 Mar 26. PMID: 33651443.

53. Babyn K, Ross S, Makowsky M, Kiang T, Yuksel N. (2023) Cannabis use for menopause in women aged 35 and over: a cross-sectional survey on usage patterns and perceptions in Alberta, Canada. BMJ Open. 2023 Jun 21;13(6):e069197. doi: 10.1136/bmjopen-2022-069197. PMID: 37344107; PMCID: PMC10314536.

Chapter 17: My Crystal Ball(s)

1. Laura Numeroff, *If You Give a Mouse a Cookie* (New York: Harper and Row, 1985).

2. "If You Give a Mouse a Cookie Summary," The Prindle Institute for Ethics, accessed October 4, 2023, https://www.prindleinstitute.org/books/if-you-give-a-mouse-a-cookie/#:~:tex-

t=Once%20the%20mouse%20is%20given,makes%20him%20want%20another%20cookie.

3. State of California, Cannabis: Local Jurisdictions: Retail Commercial Cannabis Activity Bill, CA AB 1356, California Legislature 2019-2020 Regular Session, introduced in Assembly April 4, 2019.

4. Ovetta Wiggins, "This Town Owns Part of a Weed Company. It Wants a Fair Share of The Pot," *The Washington Post*, August 22, 2023, https://www.washingtonpost.com/dc-md-va/2023/08/22/maryland-cannabis-hancock-trulieve-profits/

5. Oregon Health Authority, Marijuana and Hemp Testing, OAR 333-007, February 16, 2023, https://secure.sos.state.or.us/oard/displayDivisionRules.action?selectedDivision=1222.

6. Sophie Peel, "Oregon Court of Appeals Halts State's Aspergillus Testing Rules After Legal Challenge by Cannabis Industry," *Willamette Week*, August 25, 2023, https://www.wweek.com/news/business/2023/08/25/oregon-court-of-appeals-halts-states-aspergillus-testing-rules-after-legal-challenge-by-cannabis-industry/

7. Nate Seltenrich, "Untested, Unsafe? Cannabis Users Show Higher Lead and Cadmium Levels," *Journal of Environmental Health Perspectives* 131, no.9 (September 2023), https://doi.10.1289/EHP13519.

8. Meredith, "A Digital Tour of the Coffee Joint with Meredith," filmed September 22, 2019, The Coffee Joint, https://www.youtube.com/watch?v=6ZQJ9fPOIbA.

9. State of Colorado, Marijuana Hospitality Establishments Act, CO HB 19-1230, Colorado General Assembly 2019 Regular Session, enacted on May 29, 2019.

10. "Secondhand Marijuana Smoke," Centers for Disease Control and Prevention, last modified October 19, 2020, https://www.cdc.gov/marijuana/health-effects/second-hand-smoke.html#:~:text=THC%20can%20be%20passed%20to,effects%2C%20such%20as%20feeling%20high.

11. "Medical Marijuana Registry providers," Colorado Department of Public Health & Environment, last accessed April 20, 2023, https://cdphe.colorado.gov/medical-marijuana-registry-providers

12. Alfonso Abizaid et al. "Cannabis: A potential efficacious intervention for PTSD or simply snake oil?," *Journal of Psychiatry & Neuroscience* 44(2), (March 2019): 75-78, https://doi.org/10.1503/jpn.190021

13. NuggMD Webpage – https://www.nuggmd.com/

14. State of Oklahoma, Title 442. Oklahoma Medical Marijuana Authority, September 11, 2023, https://oklahoma.gov/content/dam/ok/en/omma/content/rules/Sept%2011%202023%20OMMA%20Emergency%20Rules.pdf

15. The Crime of the Century, "The Crime of the Century," HBO MAX video, 3:50:00, May 10, 2021, https://www.hbo.com/the-crime-of-the-century.

16. Mel Pohl, *A Day Without Pain* (Las Vegas: Central Recovery Press, 2011).

17. Mel Pohl, *The Pain Antidote* (Philadelphia: Da Capo Press, 2015).

18. "Charlie Peddie: This Epidemic Doesn't Discriminate Against Anyone," Solving SUD Together, September 5, 2023, https://solvingsudtogether.org/charlie-peddie-this-epidemic-doesnt-discriminate-against-anyone/

19. U.S. Congress, House, Secure and Fair Enforcement Banking (SAFE Banking) Act of 2023, HR 2891, 118th Cong., introduced in House April 26, 2023.

20. U.S. Congress, Senate, Secure and Fair Enforcement Regulation Banking (SAFER Banking) Act of 2023, S 2860, 118th Cong., introduced in Senate September 20, 2023.

21. Tracy Loew, "Former Eugene athletic shoe reseller among those who owe more than $50K in Oregon taxes," *The Register-Gaurd*, August 1, 2023, https://www.registerguard.com/story/news/state/2023/07/23/oregon-tax-delinquents-athletic-shoe-reseller-cannabis-entrepreneurs/70448052007/.

22. The Dab Webpage – https://www.thedab303.com/

23. Ricardo Cortés, *It's Just a Plant* (China: Akashic Books printing, 2005).

24. *2022 Monitoring the Future Panel Study Annual Report National data on substance us amount adults ages 19 to 60, 1976-2022* (Ann Arbor, University of Michigan Institute for Social Research, 2023), https://monitoringthefuture.org/wp-content/uploads/2023/07/mtfpanel2023.pdf.

25. CBS Miami, "Trulieve adds $500K to Florida recreational marijuana initiative," *CBS News*, October 11, 2023, https://www.cbsnews.com/miami/news/trulieve-adds-500k-to-florida-recreational-marijuana-initiative/.

26. CBS Miami, "Florida Attorney General Ashley Moody targets company in marijuana ballot fight," *CBS News*, August 3, 2023, https://www.cbsnews.com/miami/news/trulieve-adds-500k-to-florida-recreational-marijuana-initiative/.

27. Kwonmok Ko et al., "Psychedelic therapy for depressive symptoms: A systematic review and meta-analysis," *Journal of Affective Disorders* 322, (February 2023): 194-204, https://doi.org/10.1016/j.jad.2022.09.168.

28. Ethan Nadelmann, "Why we need to end the War on Drugs," filmed October 2014, TEDGlobal, https://www.ted.com/talks/ethan_nadelmann_why_we_need_to_end_the_war_on_drugs?language=en.

29. State of Oregon, Drug Addiction Treatment and Recovery Act (Measure 110), OR SB 755-C, Oregon State Senate 2020 Regular Session, enacted on February 1, 2021.

30. "SUDORS Dashboard: Fatal Overdose Data," Centers for Disease Control and Prevention, last modified August 25, 2023, https://www.cdc.gov/drugoverdose/fatal/dashboard/index.html.

31. "Drug Overdose Deaths," Centers for Disease Control and Prevention, last modified August 22, 2023, https://www.cdc.gov/drugoverdose/deaths/index.html.

32. *2021 Release of FBI Uniform Crime Reports for Oregon* (Oregon, Oregon Criminal Justice Commission, December 2022), https://www.oregon.gov/cjc/CJC%20Document%20Library/2021%20FBI%20UCR%20Oregon%20Report.pdf.

33. Shannon Cary, and Mark Waller, "Oregon Drug Court Cost Study: Statewide Costs and Promising Practices, Final Report," U.S Department of Justice Office of Justice Programs, March 2011, https://www.ojp.gov/ncjrs/virtual-library/abstracts/oregon-drug-court-cost-study-statewide-costs-and-promising.

www.ingramcontent.com/pod-product-compliance
Lightning Source LLC
Chambersburg PA
CBHW060909140726
47996CB00001B/181